PAIN

Dr Abdul-Ghaaliq Lalkhen has been working in pain related areas – from anaesthesiology to pain management – for over two decades. He is a member of the Faculty of Pain Medicine affiliated to the Royal College of Anaesthetists and a Visiting Professor at Manchester Metropolitan University. He lives in Manchester.

'Combines a career's worth of expertise with a long history of pain treatment. For anyone concerned with pain treatment, or anyone who has struggled to manage pain of any kind, it's an important read.' *GQ*

'As timely as it is important. What makes the book so prescient is the fact that Lalkhen understands exactly what is at stake.' *Scientific Inquirer*

'Fascinating... At some point in our life, we all hurt. This splendid book – informative, empathic, and wise – about a universal experience will surely promote healing.' *Booklist* (starred review)

'Lalkhen's mission? To change our understanding of pain so that it can be better managed... Lalkhen's genius rests in explaining the synthesis of body, mind and spirit in its manifestation... A fusion of history, psychology and science, *Pain* is a call to increase not only our level of emotional literacy but also empathy, particularly in the medical profession.' *The Australian*

'Lalkhen knows a lot about pain and how sneaky it can be. A teacher and clinician, he describes the history of pain relief: how it allows surgery, what led to the opiate crisis, how pain affects people in different ways, and how pain can outlast tissue damage... This is a book to read if you are objectively curious about how pain works.' *Listener*

PAIN

What It Is, Why It
Happens and How to Cope

Abdul-Ghaaliq Lalkhen

Atlantic Books
London

First published in hardback in Great Britain in 2021 by Atlantic Books,
an imprint of Atlantic Books Ltd.

This paperback edition first published in Great Britain in 2022
by Atlantic Books.

2 3 4 5 6 7 8 9

A CIP catalogue record for this book is available from
the British Library.

E-Book ISBN: 978-1-78649-706-2
Paperback ISBN: 978-1-78649-707-9

Printed in Great Britain by
Severn, Gloucester

Atlantic Books
An Imprint of Atlantic Books Ltd
Ormond House
26–27 Boswell Street
London
WC1N 3JZ

www.atlantic-books.co.uk

To my wife Nichola, whose patience and kindness has no equal, and to my parents and siblings who have always been both the anchors of my life and the wind in my sails.

'But pain is perfect misery, the worst of evils,
and, excessive, overturns all patience.'

John Milton, *Paradise Lost*

Contents

An unexpected journey

There is a special quality to the sound of the telephone when it rings at two in the morning. When you are working as the anaesthesiologist on a labour ward that call causes your heart to race and your stomach to do a little flip, adding another layer of fatty damage to your over-stressed coronary arteries. You have usually just fallen into an uneasy sleep on a lumpy bed in a damp but overheated on-call room, where many doctors have tossed and turned before you. The voice on the other end of the line is typically that of a harassed and overworked midwife. 'Epidural – room 4' might be all you hear before the deafening click of the slammed handset. There is the urban legend of an anaesthesiologist who, on receiving such a message, walked up to the room he had been sent to and stuck an epidural needle directly into the door before turning around and going back to his bed.

On entering a birthing room at 2.00 a.m., when the human spirit is at its lowest ebb, the scene is often predictable. There is a partner who looks scared out of his wits, a midwife who is fretting and trying her best to reassure everyone and a pregnant woman who is screaming in pain. You are greeted by an individual who would normally present a reasonable and calm image to the world but who is now reduced to a feral and illogical spectre as she is consumed with pain. The pain experienced during labour does not spare social class, colour or creed. Pain reduces us all to our barest elements; it is a great equalizer and unifier and one thing we all share an experience of.

As an anaesthesiologist you are therefore confronted by a woman who is demanding pain relief and may now be screaming at you and everybody who comes into her line of vision. Administering an epidural in these circumstances is challenging to say the least. When you return later, however, and the epidural has taken effect, you are greeted by somebody completely different – a calm, personable individual. The ability to transform someone's demeanour completely by abolishing a barrage of unpleasant sensations that are coming from distended and damaged tissues has made a lasting impression on me, and I continue to be amazed at the transformation that takes place when pain is removed.

Whilst we now accept pain relief in labour as being an absolute right – and in first-world countries epidurals are provided on demand – this was not always the case. We have vacillated over the centuries between advocating that pain should be aggressively treated, and the belief that pain is necessary and important to the curing of the condition, or an integral part of the treatment being given. Inflicting suffering was thought to sometimes be inevitable, for example in the case of amputations before the invention of anaesthesia, or when 'releasing evil humours' by blood-letting with leeches. Pain was sometimes thought to be intrinsic to the success of the therapy, a sign of the patient's vigour and helpful to their personal growth. 'Pain is weakness leaving the body' was an often-shouted phrase by my rugby coach; 'Pain is good for you; it tells you that you are still alive' was a phrase sometimes used by stressed doctors in the emergency department where I worked, when the umpteenth stab victim of the evening complained about the chest drain inserted to inflate a collapsed lung.

At one time, it was believed by priests that the pain of childbirth strengthened the bond between mother and child, reinforcing the idea of self-sacrifice inherent to motherhood, and that interfering with this pain would disrupt this maternal bond. Even in the early days of medical procedures, pain was not always seen as something that needed to be treated, largely because it was a sign of whether the patient was well and whether the treatment was working. It was only after 1800 that doctors became increasingly preoccupied with managing pain from injury or surgery, treating patients who had cancer, as well as non-cancer pain such as arthritis and migraines. When surgical anaesthesia was first introduced in the mid-nineteenth century, however, there were uncertainties expressed about the ethics of operating on an unconscious person and a concern that pain relief might retard the healing process. Priests, and some physicians, feared that its use would corrupt the individual's soul, bringing into play a moral calculator to assess whether pain should be relieved or not. The development of medicine and surgery as endeavours which can only be accomplished through relieving pain, and a philosophical shift towards the value of the individual, changed the narrative from one where pain was believed necessary and a part of human life, to it being viewed as an experience which needed to be actively managed.

Religious writers initially deemed anaesthesia in the context of childbirth a violation of God's law. This was obviously an idea proposed by men, and it was not until Queen Victoria had chloroform to facilitate the birth of one of her children that the practice of providing women with analgesia during labour achieved acceptance. Even today, the application of pain relief in labour varies across the globe; the mechanical stretching and contraction of tissues during labour is interpreted, perceived and responded to through the woman's unique social and cultural lens. In the Chinese and Korean cultures, for example, birth must appear to be pain-free and is endured in silence, in order to not bring shame to the woman's family, whereas in other cultures a more vocal response is believed to ensure a more solicitous and attentive husband.

What is it about pain that makes some people require medical intervention and others not? The storm of information created and transmitted by nerves when we are burnt, stabbed, bumped, bruised, shot, frozen, disappointed in love and life, jarred, shaken and irradiated is perceived, interpreted and modulated by our individual brains, which are as unique as snowflakes famously are. Pain, too, is therefore unique, individual and often confounds us and those we love and who love us.

*

I work at the Manchester and Salford Pain Centre at Salford Royal NHS Foundation Trust in the UK. The hospital is a major trauma and neurosciences centre located 5 km from the Manchester United football stadium. I split my time between anaesthetizing patients in the operating theatre, inserting electrical devices to relieve chronic pain and assessing individuals with chronic pain in an outpatient setting. But the reason I chose a career in anaesthetics was initially in order to become an intensive care doctor.

I was born and raised in South Africa, attending school and university under the shadow of Table Mountain. As a junior doctor in South Africa I worked in a major trauma centre and was exposed to some of the most hor- rific human-inflicted trauma imaginable. During the nine months that I spent in an inner-city trauma unit I devel- oped a deep and pervasive antipathy towards people in general, and felt that I could only survive in medicine if my patients were asleep and if my interaction with them was brief. I found myself more comfortable with patients who were uncommunicative and found the stabilization of the injured person less emotionally taxing than a biopsy-chosocial assessment of the journey that had brought them to hospital. It didn't help that at the time I was unhappily in love. This was also a time when there were influential government leaders who denied that HIV caused AIDS and when this statement was repeated to me by a patient who had been diagnosed HIV-positive and who was refusing to disclose this information to her partner, I coped by running away from home.

I went on to become an anaesthesiologist, completing my training in the UK, where I remained. Over time I specialized in pain medicine, an area that often comes under the remit of anaesthesiology, for reasons we will come to later. I now work in a pain clinic, with patients who suffer acute pain – that is to say pain with an easily identifiable cause (traumatic injury or surgery) that will eventually go away when the physical damage heals – or with chronic pain, that may not have a clear cause and may not go away.

The emotion that is primarily felt when you are faced with somebody who is in pain is extreme helplessness. In many ways pain is designed to elicit this response from others because we are social animals and one of the purposes of a visible pain experience, manifest as pain behaviours, is to encourage help from others – pain behaviours have survival value. Seeking assistance after an injury is as biologically imperative today as it was a thousand years ago. What has changed over time, however, is the place of healing and the people we seek healing from. A thousand years ago a sick person might have attended a temple to meet with a priest, since health and spiritual well-being were inextricably linked and so the priest served as both healer and spiritual guide. At an even earlier time in human history, the person consulted might have been the local medicine man, who would also have communicated with the ancestors to find answers to various afflictions. Today, we have huge biomedical temples called hospitals and networks of shamans called general practitioners, organized into a hierarchical system and monitored by professional bodies.

The nature of the interaction between doctor and patient has changed over the centuries based on our accumulated knowledge of physiology and anatomy, as well as our understanding of disease and treatments. Today, most individuals in society can understand traumatic pain without knowledge of the complex neurophysiology involved. We understand to a degree that if we injure ourselves then we experience pain, in the same way that a car or house that is broken into results in activation of an alarm. Pain is an alarm bell that something is wrong and a call to seek medical help. In the modern world, however, our understanding of pain as an alarm system has limited benefit in a society where we voluntarily subject ourselves to the trauma of surgery, for example – and yet pain continues its primitive wail despite our enhanced ability to understand and manage trauma and disease. It is this disconnect between the biological and the psychological that often makes modern pain management ineffective. Even when pain is due to an injury, seeking help is easily understood but it is still governed by the individual's perception of the severity of the injury and their health-seeking behaviour, which in turn is governed by a host of psychosocial and cultural factors. Most people, including doctors, do not appreciate that the organ which produces pain is the brain. It is not the broken bone, or the damaged tissue or the bleeding wound. The experience of pain is the sum total of more than just the physical injury – it is the result of this information being filtered through the individual's psychological make-up, genetics, gender, beliefs, expectations, motivations and their emotional context.

We have a collective delusion that the human body is a simple machine that can be repaired by the medical profession when it breaks down. However, the reality is that the human body is not a simple machine; it is an organism which progressively deteriorates over time and then, eventually, ceases to function. Pain as an experience is often seen simplistically as a manifestation of a dysfunctional machine, and is often a consequence, when it becomes chronic, of a machine that has been poorly treated. Unfortunately, rather than recognizing that it is the behaviour towards the machine that needs to change, we have a tendency to medicalize this pain and therefore often apply excessive amounts of lubrication in the form of opioids and surgery, which do nothing to improve the function of the machine and in fact can cause a significant deterioration of the organism.

Simply put, we need to stop viewing our bodies as machines that medicine can fix when they go wrong. If people are educated about their bodies and about pain, then perhaps we might put an end to the undulating fashions of medical meddling; meddling which, in some cases, has far-reaching consequences only appreciated decades later. We are currently, for example, at the tail end of an epidemic of opioid prescribing and are beginning to see the effect of that rampant scourge on individuals and on our society. Once upon a time the use of opiates was the province of recreational drug users and abstaining from opioids, even in the face of severe pain, was considered not only appropriate but admirable. The changing understanding of the possible advantages of treating pain after surgery or injury swung the pendulum towards increased opioid prescribing, with the relief of pain regarded as a human right and a benefit to the patient. We now see addiction, tolerance, dependence and withdrawal, as well as the long-term physical effects of prescription opioid use on patients. We have begun to realize, as medical professionals, that our over-zealous management of acute post-operative pain and our mistaken treatment of chronic pain (as opposed to acute pain due to injuries) with the same medication has had unintended consequences.

My mission in this book is to explain pain in all its forms – pain from physical trauma, cancer pain and pain which appears to continue in the absence of any physical damage. We all suffer with pain at some point in our lives and are witness to the pain of those we love and care for. With renewed knowledge and understanding, we can become active participants in the art of caring, understanding and coping with an experience that can become all-consuming.

How does pain work?

You may have purchased this book to read whilst on holiday somewhere, as you bask in sunshine. Currently you may be being tortured or delighted by the excited screams of children around you, or feeling gentle breezes blowing from the sea, whilst the smell of suntan oil permeates the surrounding air. Your swimsuit may be slightly damp from the last time you were in the swimming pool. Regardless of the sounds, smells and temperatures you are exposed to, these sensations are all quite easy to tune out and simply become background noise. However, if you were to be bitten by a mosquito, or an exposed part of your body started to object to the strong sunlight, then this experience would demand your attention and it would take a great deal of conscious effort to ignore. This is the universal experience of pain. Physiologists like to refer to pain as 'aversive at threshold', which means that it cannot be ignored or subdued easily. Its very nature demands attention, and this is as true today, as you sit languishing idly around a swimming pool, as it was when we were a primitive species fighting for survival in a harsh and untamed world.

But whilst damage to our bodies may eventually demand our attention through the experience of pain, this experience can be ignored, sublimated or delayed by the brain. Pain is a warning system, informing us that there is a threat to the safety of our bodies or even that damage has already occurred, but if experiencing pain and receiving this information is not immediately beneficial then the message relaying this information will be de-prioritized and sometimes ignored by the brain. We all know how crippling and all-consuming the experience of pain can be, and if it might delay, for example, our flight to safety, then it is not immediately helpful and could even be dangerous. The relationship between physical damage and the experience of pain can tell us a lot about the complexity of the biological pain alarm system and the processing of the information about damage, the route this message takes, and why, how and when it can be disrupted.

Whilst playing for Milan against Chievo on 14 March 2010, David Beckham ruptured his Achilles tendon in the eighty-ninth minute of the game. Video footage shows him turning sharply and trying to control the ball – the sharp turn is probably what caused the injury. He then starts to limp because his ankle will no longer flex and extend since he has now lost the use of his calf muscles that rely on being fixed to the ankle bones via the Achilles tendon. It appears that initially he does not realize he has injured himself – I imagine most professional sportspeople exist with a level of discomfort that would be abnormal to the rest of us and so the natural tendency would be to ignore the messages reaching his brain and carry on in the context of practising his profession. He tries again to run up to the ball to kick it but finds that he cannot perform this action – his progress is halted not by pain, as yet, but by loss of mechanical function. The tear to his Achilles tendon has already occurred moments before, and whilst the process by which information about this damage is converted to an electrical signal began at the moment of injury, it has not yet registered in his brain as pain.

When you sustain an injury, the traumatized tissue releases and attracts chemicals called inflammatory mediators. The aim of these substances is to try to heal the damaged tissue, but they also play a role in triggering the pain alarm. The release of chemicals such as hydrogen ions, potassium ions, bradykinins and prostaglandins stimulates the harm-sensing receptors in the tissues. The first step in the body's complex pain alarm system, which we all possess (unless we are born with congenital hypoalgesia, which is a condition where people do not feel pain), is the conversion of damage to the body into an electrical signal. Throughout our bodies there exist receptors (which are like locks on doors) on free nerve endings called nociceptors – the prefix *noci* means harm or mischief in Greek – and these are harm-sensing receptors. Harm-sensing nerve endings are widely distributed in the skin, muscle, joints, organs and the lining of the brain, and are either covered with myelin, which is a fatty tissue, or are uncovered. Myelin-sheathed nerve endings (A delta fibres) conduct electricity faster than their thinner uncovered counterparts (C fibres); the faster signals from the A delta fibres make you instantly remove your hand from a hot object, whereas the slower fibres produce the sensation that teaches you not to do it again.

The human body can only be injured in three ways: mechanical trauma (such as gunshots, stabs, bumps and scrapes), chemical injury (a burn from an acid or an alkaline substance) and injury from extremes of temperature. All of these injuries result in the release of inflammatory mediators. Inflammation can also occur when the body's immune system attacks itself or joints become inflamed. Nociceptors are of different classes and, like locks, they are all opened with different keys – intense pressure, temperatures greater than 40 to 45°C or less than 15°C, or chemicals released from injury and inflammation. In Beckham's case, the damaged Achilles tendon releases substances including histamine, serotonin, bradykinin and hydrogen ions, which insert themselves into nociceptors, triggering an electrical impulse which communicates and codes for harm and damage, and begins its journey to the brain, where that message can be decoded.

The information that the body has been damaged first passes from the Achilles tendon to an area of the spinal cord called the dorsal horn and information is then passed into the substance of the spinal cord, which is an extension of the brain, and enables communication between the brain and the rest of the body. The dorsal horn is constantly receiving information both from the outer reaches of the body and from the brain via the spinal cord; it is like a bowl of soup whose flavour can be altered by inputs from the brain or from the peripheral nerves, rather than existing as a hardwired, fixed computer component. The face and neck are slightly different to the rest of the body, in that the nociceptive nerve endings meet in a structure called the trigeminal ganglion which projects to the brainstem that is located in the base of the brain.

Once the thin C fibres and fat A delta fibres mentioned above have conveyed information to the first and second layers of the dorsal horn, a chemical substance called glutamate is released from the dorsal horn nerves when the electrical signal generated from nociceptor activity reaches it and this opens doors within the spinal cord, sending a message to the brain about what has happened. The graver the injury, or the more times it is inflicted, the more keys are made available and the more doors are opened, resulting in more information being sent from the spinal cord to the brain – a phenomenon called wind-up, which contributes to the persistence of pain even when the injury has healed.

There are five superhighways of information ascending to the brain from the spinal cord – the spinothalamic tract (the 'where is the problem' pathway); the spinoreticular and spinomesencephalic tracts (triggering arousal, emotion, fight or flight instincts and activating motivation circuits in the brain which determine how we behave towards injury based on previous experience); and the cervicothalamic and spinohypothalamic pathways (controlling the regulation of hormones).

From the Achilles tendon this information rushes to the brain via these superhighways in the spinal cord and lights up different parts of the brain like the colours from a single firework which when ignited spreads across the night sky. The information travels to the area of the brain called the thalamus which is connected to the sensory part of the brain which deals with location and sensation (spinothalamic), as well as the areas which are responsible for sensing and coordinating emotion (spinohypothalamic), mediating the emotional components of pain. The survival and awareness areas of the brain are reached via the spino-reticular circuit, bringing into play the areas that facilitate an increase in heart rate, blood glucose and blood pressure to deal with whatever danger may be around. Connections are also made to the parts of the brain that deal with motivation. We are driven as humans by that which is necessary for survival – food, sleep, the avoidance of pain – and we are also driven by rewards which can be any experience that facilitates learning or results in pleasure; these motivation circuits develop early on and continue developing throughout our lives, determining how we behave. The damage signals also reach the parts of the brain that can release substances which cause pain relief (naturally occurring opioids and cannabinoids). Connections are made to the pathways that descend from the brain to the spinal cord and which are responsible for suppressing signals from the spinal cord, reducing the unpleasant information reaching the brain and thereby reducing the pain experienced. Pain is therefore always a sensory and an emotional experience, as these 'superhighways' connect to areas of the brain that involve both.

What is interesting when rewatching the footage of Beckham being injured is that initially there is no indication that he is in pain – he frowns, more confused than distressed, and continues to try to play. He eventually realizes that he cannot kick the ball and examines the area of his body that is not working properly. He knows where he has been injured because his brain has already received a message from the Achilles tendon which has registered in the part of the brain that deals with location when it comes to pain, but we do not yet see his outward expression of pain because the information is still being considered and evaluated.

What follows this assessment of the injured area is the realization of the injury and, more importantly, its meaning for him as an individual. This information is then processed through the parts of his brain that deal with emotion and context (the hypothalamus). I bet his initial thought was, 'No World Cup. There goes my chance of captaining England.' Once this information has been processed by his brain, we see him collapse under the weight of the implication of this injury. He lies on the ground distraught, holding his head in his hands. We see not only the expressions of pain but also the very visible experience of suffering. The sequence of events that we have witnessed, from the moment that he struggles to strike the ball to his collapse, is a powerful example of how pain and injury are not proportional to one another. It is only when an individual processes the injury in terms of attaching meaning to it that the expressions of suffering and pain are exhibited. In this way pain is a form of communication – it allows other people to see what the injury means to us as individuals and it has survival value in that our expression of pain will produce empathy and assistance.

Beckham sits on the bench with a towel over his head. The injury has not healed and therefore harm-sensing receptors are still being activated – nociception is ongoing. The information continues to reach the parts of his brain that were activated at the time of the injury, but he is no longer rolling about on the pitch; the experience of pain has been suppressed to a degree. This is caused by the activation of descending inhibitory pathways which project from the brain down to the spinal cord. The brain, therefore, can modulate the information coming up from the injured area and the pain experience is altered. The brain acts like a policeman controlling traffic, deciding how many of the cars coming from the Achilles tendon are allowed through. The brain also decides how much attention to pay to the individual drivers of these cars. The need for immediate attention is over for Beckham – the behaviours which he exhibited are no longer necessary, nor are they socially or psychologically acceptable. The game must go on and he must retire privately to decide on where he goes from this point in his life. This is the loneliness of the pain experience.

The descending inhibitory pathways which project from the brain are poorly understood. Functional magnetic resonance imaging (fMRI), which lights up parts of the brain in response to a painful stimulus, has been used to theorize about which areas of the brain are involved in suppressing pain. Parts of the emotional centre of the brain, the hypothalamus, which is responsible for appraising the sensory information, as well as the rostroventral medulla (part of the midbrain), are important for integrating these descending pathways to the spinal cord. Interestingly the same brain chemicals which we try to increase with medication when treating depression (serotonin and noradrenaline) are fundamental to the activation and functioning of these pathways. This is why individuals who are depressed often experience increased pain, because the lower levels of these chemical neurotransmitters are insufficient to activate the descending inhibitory pathways.

And so, we see that not all signals that are being sent from the Achilles tendon are being perceived in Beckham's brain at the point of injury and in the immediate aftermath. Attention to the injury, emotional processing of the experience, expectation and thinking about the meaning of what has happened – these are all triggering return messages from the brain that regulate and control the information travelling from the injured area and moderate the consequent pain suffered.

I often use the example of David Beckham's injured tendon when I explain to medical students the difference between tissue damage and pain. Initially he does not appear to be in pain; although of course we do not know that this is the case and can only surmise from the behaviour that he exhibits. He tries to continue to play. The information about the damage has already reached his brain but until he makes sense of what has gone wrong, we would not recognize his behaviour as that of exhibiting pain. This same situation, with regards to the mental processing of an injury, is why soldiers injured in battle are sometimes not found to complain significantly of pain even in the presence of horrific injuries such as amputations. The immediate concern of the individual is to get to safety and the brain can override the pain experience to facilitate this. It is only when soldiers reach a place of safety that an appraisal of the injury can be made. The injury results in the soldier having to leave the battlefield – a place of danger – and once this stress factor is removed the individual's response to the injury similarly changes. In 1981, Ronald Reagan was shot in an attempted assassination. He recalled later that he only realized he had been shot in the chest when he felt and saw the blood seeping through his shirt in the limousine on the way to hospital.

The above examples of a delayed pain experience can be contrasted with those of people who are caught in fires, where immediate and severe pain is experienced. When you have been burnt in a civilian situation there is none of the modulating environment of a battlefield with its chaos or the distraction of being hastened to safety by Secret Service agents and nor, crucially, was there any expectation of possible injury when entering the arena and so the event is unexpected and thus deemed catastrophic by the victim. Burn injuries are also amongst the most painful given the degree of damage which is done and the widespread activation of harm-sensing receptors on nerve endings.

We all appreciate and understand the kind of pain described above, caused when tissues are broken, torn or damaged in some way; it is no different, perhaps, from the experience of primitive or ancient man, who understood the pain inflicted by an arrow, but failed to appreciate the pain from degenerative joints or infected, inflamed tissues. But as we have seen, injury and pain are not proportional, and the outcome of pain is dependent on more than just the degree of damage sustained – this can be harder to understand.

Pain as an experience is influenced by beliefs and expectations as well as psychological factors such as mood and resilience. An individual's culture, genetics and innate ability to cope with adversity will all impact on their experience of pain. The rupture of an Achilles tendon on a squash court has very different implications to the same injury in a professional footballer who has aspirations of captaining a national side in a World Cup tournament; a soldier on the battlefield responds very differently to discomfort or injury than a member of the public who is injured at home, yet they both have the same internal chemistry.

The complexity of the psychological experience of pain is often best understood by looking at an individual's reaction when they sustain an injury – their facial expressions, language and the sounds they make. But this needs to be considered alongside the physical processes taking place; the danger is that we might begin to consider the psychological experience as being separate from the pain pathways that I have described above. I talked about activation, for example, of the fight or flight system. We know that the release of adrenaline as a response to stress can cause an increase in muscle tension and the increase in muscle tension reduces blood flow (and therefore oxygen supply) to the muscle, which then releases bradykinin in response to being starved of oxygen; the bradykinin then activates more harm-sensing receptors. Anxiety and stress, therefore, which we would regard as psychological constructs, influence the pain experience on a biological basis. If a doctor is kind to you in a hospital when you are in pain, then that pain can be relieved to a degree even before the doctor has given you any pain relief, because kindness activates the descending inhibitory pathways. Similarly, whilst hostile social situations or hazardous environmental factors can cause the suppression of pain, as we saw in the instance of soldiers on a battlefield, in other environments these factors can actually aggravate the pain experience because, as we saw with adrenaline, stress influences the production of hormones, which activate parts of the brain that can either exacerbate or relieve the pain. The differing effects of psychosocial factors on an individual's pain experience depend on how they are interpreted. There is, therefore, an integral relationship between psychological, social and environmental factors with tissue injury. This is why, when considering the experience of pain, a biopsychosocial model is used, which proposes that psychological and behavioural processes are mediated by the individual's biology, rather than representing some esoteric force which descends from the ether – in other words, eventually it's all down to chemistry.

As human beings we struggle with understanding how our behaviours and thoughts influence our biology via hormones and neurotransmitter chemicals. It is why individuals with mental health disorders are so marginalized and poorly understood and are therefore discriminated against, whilst we readily accept high blood pressure as a disease because it has a physiological explanation, even if most of us would never be able to outline how blood pressure functions within our bodies. Very few individuals understand that normal blood pressure is the product of the output of the heart multiplied by the resistance in their blood vessels and that abnormal blood pressure is a result of dysfunction of these blood vessels. We would not respond to somebody with high blood pressure by telling them to calm down or relax their blood vessels. Unfortunately, patients who present with pain that we consider to be in excess of what we would expect, or who have lowered mood, are often told to just get on with it and to stop being histrionic.

*

Depression and anxiety play a role in the experience and report of pain. Catastrophizing is a psychological construct that consists of excessive rumination, magnification and helplessness in the face of adversity, and involves extreme negative thoughts about one's plight. A higher level of catastrophizing, and consequently feeling a lower sense of control, is an important predictor that a patient will experience severe acute pain or develop chronic pain, when pain persists beyond what would be medically expected. Catastrophizing may be thought of as an exaggerated negative pattern of thinking which is brought to bear during actual or anticipated painful experiences. Where patients catastrophize to a high degree they experience greater levels of pain and emotional distress. This abnormal pattern of thinking can have a significant biological impact, as it can increase pain signals and may result in increased sensitivity of the pain alarm, potentially leading to the permanent activation of the pain alarm even after the once-damaged tissues have healed and resulting in progression from acute to chronic pain.

This can be in part due to the development of pain-related fear, where patients adopt an approach to managing persistent pain by trying to avoid activities that might cause an increase in pain. Patients who have undergone surgery or experienced trauma and who have high levels of catastrophizing, for example, may find it difficult to rehabilitate because of this psychological construct. Their way of coping with pain is to avoid movement; however, this may have consequences such as the development of deep vein thrombosis when they remain in bed and the blood in their legs pools like stagnant water, as well as lung infections when they fail to cough or breathe deeply following surgery. These patients are also more likely to use higher doses of pain-relief medication.

Preoperative anxiety is one of the most consistent and predictable risk factors for the severity of post-operative pain. One of the key messages that I communicate to trainee doctors who assess patients prior to surgery is to never tell anybody that they will have no pain following surgery. I tell them to explain to the patient that if zero equals no pain and ten is the worst pain imaginable, then at best we can probably get their pain down to four following the operation. If patients have this 4/10 construct in their heads when they wake up and assess the sensory information reaching their brain, then it may allow them to cope better with the post-operative pain. If you tell them that they will feel *no* pain when they wake up, then any unpleasant sensory information will be appraised in a catastrophic manner.

The importance of this approach is often emphasized to me when I look after patients who have had a laparotomy, which involves cutting through all of the individual's abdominal muscles and tissues to get to their bowels. The incision is often 10 or 15 cm long and can extend from above the pubic bone to just below the chest. We use epidural pain relief for these operations, and this is often very successful; a catheter is threaded into the epidural space, which lies just above the spinal cord, and the infused local anaesthetic bathes the nerves as they leave the spine. This technique usually provides excellent pain relief for what is a massive traumatic incision. These operations often require patients to have a plastic tube in their throats for a prolonged period and also to have a plastic drip put into one of their neck veins. I am always amazed when patients wake up and complain bitterly of the plastic tube in their neck and a sore throat, and are almost unmanageable as a consequence, in the face of a 15-cm incision which is being covered from a pain relief point of view by the epidural. The anaesthesiologists' preoccupation with the laparotomy wounds and the epidural often causes us to forget that patients will attach meaning to *any* unpleasant sensory information following surgery, even for issues that we would regard as minor compared with the pain that they would be experiencing if they did not have the epidural. This is why patient-centred care is much more successful in helping people than clinician-centred care.

The idea that patients would expect to not feel any abnormal sensations after surgery confuses doctors and nurses who work in the healthcare setting on a daily basis, as people who have been trained in the use of analgesics appreciate quite readily that these medications cannot abolish pain completely. I think that it sometimes doesn't occur to health-care workers that, whilst over time we have become rooted within a culture that understands a vast amount about how the human body functions, even now our understanding is sometimes imperfect. When I teach neurosurgeons, for example, I point out to them that when they look at their hands what they see are structures that all have names and nerves that provide sensation to specific areas of the hand that they give sensation to. They understand how tendons make fingers move and how those structures are often located in the forearm. It is therefore not surprising to them that if a nerve is damaged at the elbow then the function of the hand is affected. Most laypeople, however, have a more rudimentary understanding of how their bodies function, with beliefs that are often more fixed in urban legend than science, in the same way that the petrol engine or the inner workings of a computer are a mystery to me. It is therefore our privilege and responsibility as healthcare professionals to engage with the patient and to try to translate medical information into imagery and language that paints a lucid picture. I think sometimes that, just as there is a Professor of the Public Translation of Philosophy at some universities, there should exist a faculty for training individuals who aim to bridge the chasm between the science of medicine and its intended beneficiaries. Unfortunately, the belief is that this is done naturally by doctors.

Whilst patients may not need to understand the detail of the named circuits and molecules involved in producing the experience of pain, as we have described in this chapter, it is important that they understand how powerfully the interpretation of what they are feeling impacts on the pain experienced for any given injury. An understanding of the role of thoughts and feelings will enable the person suffering to be able to manage their expectations regarding pain and its management. Whilst the distress associated with the pain experience is normal and often useful in that it can provide crucial information and lead an individual to seek the appropriate help, a good understanding of what influences pain and why can be hugely beneficial in both managing pain and even decreasing it (by reducing feelings of being overwhelmed and distressed), as we have explored. Pain is, after all, both a sensory and an emotional experience, with the initial information regarding the damage activating various different parts of the brain and triggering a complex physiological and psychological response. It is only by addressing the complete experience of pain that we can hope to manage pain and alleviate suffering.

A brief history of pain

The historical record indicates that pain has always been a part of human existence and any organism which has consciousness will be subject to it. The experience of pain is primal and facilitates avoidance and education about situations that could lead to the end of our existence. Parchment scrolls from Ancient Greece and inscriptions on Babylonian clay tablets, as well as papyri written in the days when the pharaohs ruled Egypt, testify to the fact that human beings have long been preoccupied with understanding and extinguishing pain.

Historically, in the absence of an understanding of the physiology and mechanism of pain perception we resorted, as humans always do, to creating meaning and learning from experience. It was possibly very easily discovered by primitive mankind that if they rubbed an injured part of their body it reduced pain, or if the injured limb was exposed to an alternative stimulus, such as cold water or the heat of the sun, that pain could also be alleviated. Today, we take for granted a basic understanding of human anatomy and physiology, even amongst laypeople, but to primitive man pain from internal disease must have seemed quite disturbing. As a result, narratives and explanations were formulated and invented to understand the experience of pain in the same way that creation myths sought to explain the origins of man and his purpose on Earth in the absence of our current scientific language.

In primitive societies the intrusion of evil spirits, demons or magic fluids were often regarded as the reason why people experienced pain – the aversive nature of the pain experience coupled with a lack of diagnostic tests to identify its cause is perhaps the reason why pain was regarded as evil and demonic. Pain management in these early days therefore involved warding off evil spirits using tattoos, amulets and talismans derived from animals.

Primitive man also experimented with various herbs and plant foods which were found serendipitously to relieve pain. It is thought, for example, that intestinal parasites were treated by prehistoric alpine North Europeans with a birch polypore fungus (the fungus was discovered on a 5300-year-old mummy in the Italian Alps who was found to have intestinal parasites that the fungus actively attacks). At the more extreme end it has been speculated that Peruvians used trepanning (making a hole in your skull to enable a spirit causing your pain to leave) as early as 400 BC to treat headaches or epilepsy, which has been identified as the first surgical procedure. This would make neurosurgery the most ancient of surgical practices and, as I like to remind the neurosurgeons I encounter, makes them truly prehistoric in their dispositions. When contact was made with Aboriginal tribes of central and southern Australia in the late nineteenth century it was found that broken bones were set by Aborigines using clay and that wounds were covered with animal fat and bound with bark or animal skin. We still exhibit elements of this primitive behaviour today, when we employ traditional treatments in the form of warming rubs, cod liver oil and home remedies to relieve pain. These have no empirical basis but reside in the collective cultural memory.

When we reach the end of our homespun therapies, we often resort to someone who represents comfort – in my case usually my mother, even though my dad is a GP, or a wise aunt. The first healers, according to anthropologists, were women, who were viewed as representing the wide-bosomed Gaia or great Earth mother and acted as both priestesses and sorceresses. Given that women were the conduits of life in the form of the birth process they were seen as being more connected to human suffering and therefore better equipped to help alleviate it. As in most cultures and throughout recorded time, whenever women have originated an industry, men will take control if they feel that power or money can be made from it, and over time the medicine man took over from the medicine woman as the magician responsible for driving out demons. At this stage in history, 'medicine' referred less to the administering of physical substances and more to spiritual healing.

In Ancient Egypt (around 4000 BC), painful conditions that stemmed from something other than a physical wound were deemed to be caused by the influence of gods or by spirits of the dead which entered the person through their nostrils or their ears whilst they were sleeping. By vomiting, sneezing or sweating these demons could be extruded. Even today, despite our advanced understanding of viruses, we are still told not to sit on cold floors or we will 'catch cold' or that the source of an upper respiratory tract infection is due to walking outside without a coat rather than the transmission of a virus through secretions. Whilst we don't call the resultant infection a demonic possession our language nevertheless does not incorporate a modern understanding of why we are afflicted, and the causal relationship is therefore more imagined than real.

The Egyptians also developed the first neurophysiological explanation for pain, describing a fluid network which ran throughout the body carrying the essence of life and sensations. They understood that blocking the River Nile resulted in poor crops and this idea was applied to people; for example, berries of the castor oil tree (a laxative) were used to facilitate unblocking when people were unwell or in pain. The Egyptians had an extensive pharmacopoeia, including the use of honey as a medicine to heal infected wounds because of its antibacterial properties – not understood scientifically by the Egyptians at the time but appreciated practically – and surgery and dentistry were well developed. Simple surgery such as circumcision of male children was the norm, because of the belief that it was cleaner to be circumcised.

The Babylonians, some 2000 years later, worked on a similar system which saw religion and early medicine run hand in hand. They often used incantations, akin to prayers, in their treatments to relieve pain since the society was organized around religion – Babylon means 'Gateway of the Gods' – and the gods were believed to decide all matters dealing with human fate, including those of health or sickness. Demons were considered to be the invisible bearers of disease, making banishing afflictions a religious affair. The role of priest and physician was therefore rolled into one – 'it's the will of the Gods' becoming a useful explanation for pain.

The work of these early healers often involved changing the physical attributes of both his person (think white coat and stethoscope) as well as his place of residence (think hospitals) in order to exorcize demons and ritualize or formalize the experience; an illness thought to have a spiritual cause could only be cured in a spiritual place. Belief in a therapy, and the subsequent creation of a profession, is often aided by a specific location for the work of the professional, causing a powerful placebo effect through setting the process apart from daily life, endowing it with a certain status and embedding it within the meaning and beliefs of the society and the individual. The advent of agrarian societies – therefore settled as opposed to nomadic – resulted in ever more elaborate hospitals/religious edifices. Healing and religion became more complex given that more people were needed to run these places, with the inevitable production of hierarchies.

There may have been religious underpinnings to the Ancient Babylonian medical system, but it was a profession nonetheless, and was policed accordingly. The fee structure for medical services was divided into a public (slaves) and private (non-slaves) system with a reduced fee for slaves. According to King Hammurabi's code for medical practitioners, if a slave died during surgery the doctor had to replace him with another slave; if you killed a private patient your hands were cut off.

The Ancient Chinese focused on the imbalance between Yin and Yang as the cause for illness and pain, mentioned in records as early as 771 BC but the concepts of which can be traced much further back to the Shang Dynasty around 1100 BC. Traditional concepts such as Yin and Yang have been integrated alongside modern medical thinking in the People's Republic of China, a process which began in the 1950s. In a normal person Yin, which is a feminine and passive force (also regarded as cold and damp and representing the lower body), is balanced by Yang, which is the positive active force (upper part of the body and back, warm and dry). The vital energy called the Qi circulates to all parts of a network consisting of fourteen channels or 'meridians' which are connected to the internal organs and their functions. A deficiency or an excess in the circulation results in an imbalance between Yin and Yang with consequent illness. If there is free flow of Qi, there is no pain; if there is no free flow, there is pain. Acupuncture, which places needles at various points along these meridians, corrects the imbalance by redirecting the flow of Qi and therefore eliminates pain and disease. Importantly there is no differentiation when it comes to treating psychological versus physical disease in the Chinese system, as both are due to an imbalance in Qi.

As well as acupuncture, the Ancient Chinese had a pharmacopoeia of over 100,000 substances ranging from animal matter to human body parts. Research into traditional Chinese medicines, many of which are still used today, has often been critical because of a lack of a defined mechanism of action and the toxicity associated with some of the treatments. The use of substances derived from endangered species has also been criticized. Pharmaceutical research has yielded few useful therapies, however proponents of traditional Chinese medicine have indicated that complex interactions between medicines have been passed over, accounting for the lack of effectiveness found.

In India, Ayurvedic medicine can be traced back as far as 800 BC. The word 'Ayurveda' translates as 'the science of life' or 'longevity'. Within this practice concepts of disease are related to imbalances in the three *doshas* (*vata*, *pitta* and *kapha*); for example, pain is the characteristic feature of deranged *vata*. The Buddha attributed the universality of pain in life to the fulfilment (or lack thereof) of desires and remarked that any absence or separation of pleasure resulted in pain, a theory that was later echoed in Greek thought by the philosopher Plato. In the absence of an understanding of neurophysiology and in a society seeking meaning through religious belief, the emotional component of pain was given much more attention than its sensory component or physical cause. The Buddha is often quoted as having said that pain is inevitable, but that suffering is optional. In recent times, we have all but reversed this prioritization. There is an increasing realization in our modern societies that our pursuit of a material, scientific paradigm has left us turning towards nihilism or acceptance of inflexible authoritarian structures. Our medical science is not always as helpful as we would like to believe, and when it fails us we no longer have the emotionally comforting meaning-making mythologies of Ancient China, India or Egypt to fall back on.

Our word for 'pain' similarly has a combined religious and sociological etymology. It comes from the Greek word for penalty, *poine*, and the Latin word *poena* meaning punishment, but Poena was also the name given to the Roman spirit of vengeance and the attendant of Nemesis, the goddess of divine retribution. For both the Romans and the Greeks the experience of pain was laden with an emotional construct. The Greeks in particular understood the sensory and emotional nature of the pain experience and in the absence of a sound knowledge of neurophysiology emphasized the emotional aspects of this experience, much like the Ancient Egyptians and Chinese, but this was coupled with what might be considered an early scientific approach. Plato, in the fifth century BC, saw pain as both physical and emotional. He believed that human beings experienced sensation as a result of atoms moving from the veins to the heart and the liver, but that pain was not just caused by stimulation from a peripheral source, it was also an emotional experience in the soul, which was believed at the time to reside in the heart. Around half a century later, the Greek physician Hippocrates, often called the 'father of Western medicine', said 'Divine is the work to subdue pain', but his body of work also sought to find physical rather than divine origins for pain and disease.

It was the Greeks who first proposed that the brain was the centre for sensation and reason. This view, however, did not gain widespread acceptance, particularly since the influential philosopher Aristotle, like Plato, regarded the heart as the centre of all sensation – the capacity for pleasure was in the blood of the heart, which was also the location of the soul. Pain was similarly regarded as a quality or passion of the soul and the experience was considered as being opposite to pleasure and the epitome of unpleasantness. The ideas of Aristotle still hold sway in the world today because we talk about a broken heart when it comes to emotional distress and pain, rather than a broken brain. When we are in pain or emotionally upset what we feel most is a racing heart rather than a racing brain. The heart is a singularly impressive organ whilst the brain merely looks like a grey gelatinous mass. It is therefore quite easy to see how the narrative of pain and sensation in general became situated within the beating heart.

The Greeks developed a theory of disease which involved bodily imbalances akin to the Chinese system of Yin and Yang and the Ayurvedic system of *doshas*. In the case of the Greeks it was four humours: blood, phlegm, yellow bile and black bile. If these substances were in excess or deficit then this was the cause of illness and pain. Diseases were treated by attempting to restore balance (*eucrasia*) between the humours, often through purging, using emetics or blood-letting. This idea of the bodily humours proved enduring and was included in the Unani school of medicine in Persian and Arabic societies and persisted in various forms across Europe up until the sixteenth century when it was challenged by the Flemish physician Andreas Vesalius.

The Greeks and Romans made inroads into the burgeoning fields of physiology and medicine. In the second century AD, the Roman writer Celsus, known for his work *De Medicina* (*On Medicine*), related pain to the experience of inflammation, highlighting redness, swelling and heat as important components of this process. A contemporary of his, Aelius Galenus (known today as Galen), who was educated in Greece and Alexandria and who settled in Rome, was the court physician to Marcus Aurelius and carried out extensive experiments on dogs by tying off various bits of their nervous system and observing the consequent disability. Galen divided the body into a complex network of sensations which involved soft nerves, hard nerves and pain sensation. Pain sensation was regarded as the lowest form of sensibility. Despite Galen's contribution with regards to delineating the nervous system, Aristotle's concept of pain as passion of the soul would still prevail for twenty-three centuries.

The idea that the heart was the centre of sensation was still widely accepted by the time of the Renaissance, but had begun to be questioned because of the discrepancies between the work of Aristotle and Galen. The fall of the Byzantine Empire lead to the influx of Greek texts and their interpretation by Islamic scholars into Western Europe. The idea that the heart was merely a pump was brought about as a consequence of extensive dissection of cadavers (prohibited to Galen by Roman law, although the dissection of animals was permitted) and enabled the brain to be reassessed as the seat of sensation.

In the seventeenth century René Descartes, who was an adherent of Galen's thoughts on physiology, considered the brain and not the heart to be the centre of sensation. Descartes envisioned a single tube running from the foot to the brain which when stimulated by a large fire produced a large pain and when stimulated by a small fire produced a small pain. This was a radical departure from the idea of humours, *doshas* and the Aristotelean idea of the heart as the *sensorium commune*, the seat of all sensation. This Cartesian philosophy, which divorced sensation and emotion, has produced no end of problems, and even today pain is mistakenly considered by many healthcare professionals and patients as having to be proportional to the degree of tissue injury. Furthermore, the modern idea that pain is influenced by psychosocial factors, and by the descending and ascending facilitatory and inhibitory pathways, are still disputed and are not understood by many doctors today. There are many times when I have had to explain to a spinal surgeon why it is that after having performed the same operation for the same disease a patient's complaint of pain differs from the previous patient. It is extraordinary how a 400-year-old idea can persist in the face of overwhelming evidence.

Aristotle had described nerves in his book *De Anima* as being controlled by and originating in the heart. The word nerve in Greek meant sinew and it is easy to see how a nerve and structures such as ligaments and tendons, which link to muscles, can be mistaken for the same (something I often did as a medical student during exams where we had to identify coloured pins stuck in structures in cadavers). Galen, who criticized opinions on anatomy that were derived without dissection, recognized the spinal cord as an extension of the brain and documented that nerves controlled sensation and movement. He thought of nerves as hollow tubes through which the body's vitality (*anima spiritus*) travelled. 'White, soft, pliant and difficult to tear' was the description of nerves put forward by Avicenna (also known as Ibn Sina), a Persian physician in the early eleventh century. Alessandro Benedetti, Surgeon General of the Venetian army in 1497, described the senses as being distributed by means of the nerves like the roots of a tree.

Dissection of nerves revealed them not to have a cavity as expounded by Descartes, but there was no satisfactory alternative explanation for how they worked until the late eighteenth century when connections were made between the experiments with electricity and the function of nerves. Luigi Galvani – philosopher, physician and physicist – described the role of electricity in the nerves of dissected frogs in 1791 and Henri Milne-Edwards, a French physician and zoologist, conceptualized the body as a factory with different physiological systems having different functions; the language of science often takes on the zeitgeist of the time. The development and refining of the microscope (first invented in 1590) and the use of silver chromate to stain nervous tissue in 1873 aided the understanding of the structure and function of nerves. During the nineteenth century, physiology emerged as an experimental science with the publication in 1838 of the concept that all living things were composed of cells and the idea of homeostasis (the maintenance of internal balance of physiological processes such as temperature regulation and breathing).

The development of physiology as a scientific discipline resulted in theories about pain transmission and perception based on neurophysiological studies. The specificity theory (1859), in which pain had its own sensing apparatus (which is why it is called *specific* rather than being an intense form of touch, which we will explore in the intensive theory below), had been posited as early as the second century by Galen and picked up throughout the centuries, notably by Avicenna and Descartes. In the nineteenth century this theory was tested by selectively destroying parts of the nervous system in order to see which sensibilities were affected. This was the foundation of neuroscience, although today, with tools such as electron microscopy and functional neuroimaging, modern neuroscience embraces a more complex approach, encompassing molecular biology, computational neuroscience and electrophysiology. One can, for example, label specific red blood cells and track them, imaging in real time the different connections made in the brain's of individuals who have chronic pain versus those without when subjected to a standard stimulus or distraction techniques, thereby outlining the specific neural circuits that are altered in pain states.

The intensive or summation theory (1895), which was Aristotelian in its origin, implied that pain was the result of excessive stimulation of the sense of touch. By the end of the nineteenth century, there was conflict between the *specific* and *intensive* theories because they proposed different sensing mechanisms for pain (a specific apparatus versus an overstimulation of touch), both of which moved away from and de-emphasized the traditional Aristotelian concept that pain was an emotional experience. In 1906 the neurophysiologist Charles Sherrington discovered the receptor present on free nerve endings – the nociceptor which transduces the injury into an electrical signal and which therefore laid the argument to rest: specificity won.

The emotional component of the pain experience was supported and espoused by philosophers and psychologists well into the nineteenth century, but not by scientists. It is interesting to note that as we become scientifically more advanced and ostensibly rational, we tend to separate the emotional from that which we can measure and scientifically study. This continues today in terms of clinical practice, where the emotional component of the experience of pain is neglected in preference to being able to study receptors and pathways and abnormal structures. In clinical practice there is still an uneasy relationship between the work of pain management psychologists and those of physicians.

Theories on the system behind the experience of pain continued to abound as the century progressed. The pattern theory of pain in 1929 suggested that pain is produced by intense stimulation of non-specific receptors rather than a specific nerve for pain. The central summation theory in 1949 was an offshoot of the older summation theory and stated that intensive stimulation from nerve damage activated nerves in the spinal cord that reverberate, triggering the periphery nerves once again and causing a closed loop. The 'fourth theory of pain' introduced by James Hardy, Harold Wolff and Helen Goodell in the 1940s tried to reintroduce psychological factors within the specificity theory. They tried to communicate that pain is a combination of perception and reaction – a complex physiopsychological response which involved cognition as well as past experience, culture and psychological factors. They used this information to explain why people have different pain thresholds and why Descartes' model of commensurate pain to injury was inadequate. The sensory interaction theory (1959) proposed that there were two systems involved in the transmission of pain and other sensory information: a slow system and a fast system. Interaction between the different fibres was thought to be the reason why pain is experienced. This theory correctly identified the different nerve fibre elements of the pain alarm, but not how it works.

It was first recognized in the Second World War that individuals who are injured in a military setting often experience much less severe pain than those injured in a civilian setting. Doctors realized that there must be modulation of the sensory information that is transmitted to the brain at the level of the spinal cord, and that this modulation must be initiated by the brain, to produce different pain experiences. This would grow into the gate control theory that Ronald Melzack and Patrick Wall proposed in their paper entitled 'Pain mechanisms: A new theory' (published in *Science* in 1965) and which is still not recognized by most patients and doctors today, who instead still hold on to Cartesian theories of pain that are 400 years old.

In the 1950s Ronald Melzack and Patrick Wall proposed that the specificity theory was supported by evidence of a specialized apparatus within the nervous system for the experience of pain, but there was not a direct line-labelled pathway from periphery to brain – it was not the hollow tube proposed by Descartes nor a simple uninterrupted electrical cable. They suggested that there must be something at the level of the spinal cord itself that influences neural activity. They therefore proposed in 1965 that there is physiological specialization of the apparatus communicating harmful information and that this information is gathered, made sense of and changed at the level of the spinal cord, and is also influenced by descending pathways from the brain which are the psychological factors important in pain. This is now commonly referred to as the gate control theory, whereby an electrical impulse triggered by some form of harm can be modulated at the level of the spinal cord by a non-harmful stimulus. So, for example, if you bump your leg, triggering a pain impulse, rubbing that part of the body will then cause the activation of another nerve fibre which competes with the initial pain signal for access to the brain.

In Western industrialized societies there is a tendency to divorce the emotional component of the pain experience from the physical, reducing pain down to a dualistic Cartesian view where the mind and the body are separate, where we exist as an animal with physical processes and a psychological being outside of us, which is ethereal and esoteric. This is why we have difficulty understanding pain in the absence of tissue damage and why we also struggle to understand diseases such as depression or psychosis, which are due to dysfunctional brain neurotransmitters, but which our current medical technology (MRI scans, blood tests, ECGs, etc.) cannot definitively measure. It is therefore also difficult for people to understand why a small injury can produce significant pain because in a Cartesian world, where mind and body are separate, a small injury should produce a small pain and a large injury should produce a proportionally greater amount of pain. We therefore fail to appreciate the emotional aspect of the pain experience and the ability of the brain to amplify or diminish the signals initially produced by the injured tissue.

For most of humanity's history, pain has been considered an inevitable consequence of existence and it was therefore the meaning of the pain, rather than whether you had pain or not, which mattered. The nineteenth century, with its increasingly scientific and industrialized society, saw a shift in this view to one where individual pleasure or pain became increasingly important, bringing about a change in the way pain was viewed. Despite advances in the understanding of how the human body worked and, crucially, how it could be repaired when problems arose, the experience of pain was still a significant barrier to performing more intricate surgery. With the demonstration of anaesthesia for a dental procedure in October 1846 by William T. G. Morton it became possible to reduce the experience of pain and therefore perform more invasive operations. The use of chloroform during childbirth by James Young Simpson in 1848 potentially revolutionized obstetric care.

It may seem strange to us today, as previously mentioned, that there was a lot of debate in Europe with regards to whether or not it was ethical to operate on an unconscious patient, but we must bear in mind that the state of unconsciousness induced under anaesthesia was not well understood at the time, nor was it known what long-term effects it might have on the individual's mental process. Whilst there were once questions as to whether we even *should* treat pain, in modern times we have moved dramatically towards aggressively managing pain. Whilst the Royal College of Anaesthetists still takes the words of Hippocrates as its motto – 'It is divine to alleviate pain' – it is possible that, whilst our scientific techniques and processes have moved on, we have in fact lost sight of the bigger pictures that Hippocrates himself understood two millennia ago – that alleviating pain involves more than simply treating the body.

Give me something for the pain...

Because pain has been our constant companion throughout history, the pursuit of relief from pain and suffering has also been relentlessly chased and our treatments for pain have always been influenced by our politics, culture, available technology, scientific understanding and the meaning attached to pain.

Every autumn for the last five years, at the beginning of October, I have made the journey to the central campus of the University of Manchester to lecture the second-year medical students on pain management. This is no small task. My lecture takes the students through the management of acute and chronic pain, aims to cover the action of local anaesthetics and other analgesics using examples of the different classes of drugs, and demonstrates the key components of the biopsychosocial model of pain. I have sixty minutes to cover the breadth of my specialty, including an introduction which serves to outline where pain medicine fits into the pantheon of medical specialties.

Pain medicine sits uncomfortably amid the subspecialties of anaesthesiology. Most other anaesthesiologists can't quite understand our choice to be pain physicians (to see distressed patients and sit in clinics) and question our motives (the desire for lucrative private practice, an inability to focus, too much imagination). Sometimes we are perceived as helpful, when inserting difficult-to-place epidurals and when offering advice on complex pain patients in the preoperative setting, but we are also viewed with suspicion and curiosity because we choose to work with a group of patients that most anaesthesiologists try to avoid. We also perhaps have a different perspective to those anaesthesiologists who spend all their time in theatre – a greater appreciation of running a service and more familiarity with patient complaints – and so we usually cause anxiety at department clinical governance meetings by challenging the sometimes narrow viewpoint of our anaesthesiology colleagues.

Pain medicine is the only subspecialty of anaesthesiology which has outpatient clinics as a norm. The skill set required to work in pain medicine therefore departs radically from that of the mainstream discipline of anaesthesiology, such as developing the ability to actively listen and withstand the emotional onslaught of prolonged engagement with highly distressed individuals. Doctors working in pain clinics need to be able to empathize with patients and manage conflict, disappointment and expectations effectively. And this extends beyond patient relationships; a life spent working in pain medicine involves nurturing the capacity to work in a collaborative fashion with allied healthcare professionals in the form of physiotherapists and psychologists as well as developing meaningful relationships with GPs in the community.

Pain is, unfortunately and at great cost to both doctor and patient, merely seen as a symptom by many doctors – a means to formulating a biomedical diagnosis rather than an end or a focus in itself. I have repeatedly emphasized that pain is an experience; it is an experience of feeling unpleasant sensations from your body, sensations that are interpreted by multiple areas of the brain, areas that are responsible not just for registering sensation but for the way you think and feel. Processing abnormal feelings, either physical or emotional, makes us distressed, anxious and depressed. The pain of a broken heart is therefore no less distressing to us than that of a broken leg. Unfortunately, the way we think about pain, the medicalization of it and whether doctors feel that it should be treated or not, influences how we behave towards those abnormal sensations and the action that is then taken, or is not taken, to alleviate them.

As our scientific understanding and technology progresses, we perform more and more complex and invasive surgeries, and we demand and require the patient to cooperate from a psychological point of view with these insults. People generally don't have the ability to self-hypnotize and inhibit the sensations coming from a surgeon slicing through the sternum (the use of hypnosis to perform a chest incision has been described in scientific publications) in order to perform open heart surgery, nor do they have the ability afterwards to rationally understand that the sensations coming from the sternum that has been sliced open are perfectly acceptable because the aim was to help pump blood around their heart. We therefore must resort to medications that can enable the person to undergo these procedures, using anaesthetic agents that come in gas or liquid form, such as propofol, to make them completely unaware of what is happening. We can use medications such as local anaesthetics to block any sensation reaching your brain, both for the surgical procedure and for pain management post-operatively. We use opiate medications post-operatively because they affect the way that you interpret the sensations from your body: they make you care less. Opiates have been called the perfect 'whatever' medication because they allow you to ignore the messages that are coming from your body.

One can make a logical argument that the purpose of pain is somewhat superfluous in the context of controlled trauma, such as an operation. The biological purpose of pain is to alert the organism that harm has occurred, because if the damage was ignored then the open wound would become a conduit for infection which can lead to death. It could be argued therefore that if you consent to the trauma in advance then the pain alarm serves no purpose because you are completely aware of why you have been injured. Consenting to elective surgery is essentially consenting to having a surgeon cut through your skin, tissues and bones.

The primitive nature of the alarm, however, means that regardless of how cognitively aware you are of why you have sustained trauma, it still goes off. When treating pain we therefore try to tackle the different processes of the pain experience as explained in Chapter One: where the tissue is damaged (transduction), the network sending the signals of pain to the brain (transmission), the brain itself (perception) and the pathways that can put the brakes on excitable pain nerves (modulation). There are a number of ways that we can do this, the most common, and most frequently requested, is through the prescription of various drugs.

Before talking about drugs, it is worth mentioning that there are psychological techniques in the preoperative setting that can be used to help patients with the management of pain. Knee schools have arisen to facilitate improved pain relief and better outcomes from knee replacement surgery; these prehabilitation schools involve teaching patients about the fact that even though their knee has been successfully replaced they will still have some pain after the surgery, but that the pain is not an indication that the surgery has been unsuccessful. This facilitates rehabilitation by 'normalizing' the post-operative abnormal sensations from the knee, and patients have been found to have an increased ability to mobilize post-operatively when furnished with this information. Patients sometimes compete with one another to see who can mobilize quicker. There is no magical pharmacological therapy which has been administered – it is merely the change in perception and the management of expectations that facilitate an enhancement of the individual's recovery.

When I talk about using medication to manage pain before, during and after surgery (referred to as the acute perioperative setting) or in the management of chronic pain, I emphasize to the medical students that there is no drug in our current armoury that will completely abolish the experience of pain – apart from local anaesthetics that can *temporarily* block all transmission of electrical signals. Local anaesthetics are not suitable for long-term use, however; they are limited in terms of their duration of action when administered as a single injection and require ongoing infusions where plastic tubes need to be placed near nerves to facilitate prolonged use. These infusion devices present a conduit for infection and therefore they are limited in terms of how long they can be used. Beyond local anaesthetics, every other pain-relieving medication will not stop all the electrical signals to the brain triggered by chemical, mechanical or thermal damage. Regardless of how much or how little information is transmitted, the information that does get through will be perceived and interpreted through the unique expectations, beliefs, mood and previous experience of an individual. I therefore urge the medical students to always attempt to manage the expectations of the patient with regards to the degree of pain relief that an analgesic will facilitate.

The same principle applies to the pharmacological management of pain in either the perioperative setting, where someone has had trauma or is about to have elective surgery, or when someone suffers with chronic pain. Patients may have the expectation that following surgery they will have no pain, although this expectation may not be voiced, and when the patient does wake up with uncomfortable and abnormal sensations, which they then interpret as pain, their immediate perception is that the surgery has not gone to plan and that something is desperately wrong. Failure to communicate that the individual will feel these sensations following surgery in a patient who is anxious or catastrophizes will lead to a poor perioperative pain experience, and can undermine even the best placed thoracic epidural or judicious use of pain medication. Expectation management around the use of pharmacological agents which do not completely abolish pain following trauma or surgery is therefore fundamental.

*

The anaesthesiologist is the forgotten person in the surgical drama, quietly assessing your risk of having major surgery, optimizing the function of organs preoperatively with fluids and medications, obliterating awareness of the sound of a bone saw and ensuring your comfort following the operation. But most people only remember the surgeon.

The management of pain is one of the primary canons of the triad that makes up anaesthetic practice – the second is ensuring a lack of awareness or recall of the surgeon slicing through the tissues, and the third is muscle relaxation, because cavities must be entered that require the protective muscles to be split, such as the abdomen. Muscle relaxation is not always required, but what is fundamentally essential is the management of pain in the perioperative setting. If somebody is asleep or anaesthetized, then they cannot experience pain, which requires consciousness; the body, however, will still react to tissue damage and the physiological response to injury is seen, for example, in an increase in heart rate and blood pressure, which can in turn lead to an alteration in the patient's state of consciousness. The cutting of skin, bone and muscle may be accompanied by changes in their level of consciousness versus the depth of the anaesthetic risking accidental awareness. If they have intra-operative excitation of the nervous system from tissue injury then they may become aware of their surroundings as their level of consciousness changes due to the stimulus, which is a disaster if they are paralysed and unable to move or communicate what they are feeling. Anaesthesiologists administer pain medication intra-operatively in order to reduce this neurological excitability and also to ensure that the person is as comfortable in the post-operative setting as they can be.

You can have an operation whilst awake, using local anaesthetic to block the transmission of information. The only naturally occurring local anaesthetic is cocaine, which was known amongst Peruvians to cause numbing of the mouth and was introduced to the West in the latter half of the 1800s, where it was first used in a medical setting for an eye operation. The synthetic drug procaine (marketed under the trade name Novocain) is related to cocaine but is much less toxic and was formulated in 1904, shortly followed by lidocaine, which was developed in 1943 and came to market in 1947 as a local anaesthetic less likely to produce hypersensitivity reactions. Lidocaine is still a commonly used local anaesthetic agent today, along with bupivacaine, another member of the cocaine family.

When operating on a conscious patient, a needle can be inserted near a large nerve, surrounding it with injected local anaesthetic which will provide pain relief for around eight hours or so. The local anaesthetic crosses the membrane of the nerve and blocks the sodium channel of the nerve from the inside which means it cannot fire for as long as the local anaesthetic sits there like an unwelcome guest. Unfortunately, the needle can also inadvertently puncture the nerve, damaging it permanently and causing neuropathic pain for the rest of the patient's life, although this occurrence is rare.

Ultrasound has become the chief means by which we aim to deposit local anaesthetic safely around nerves by visualizing the tip of the needle, preventing it, theoretically, from going in too far and injuring the nerve. Ultrasound images, however, often look like black and white impressionist paintings and so nerves which are supposed to look like a bunch of grapes in cross section are sometimes not clearly seen. Anaesthesiologists like new toys and are very keen exponents of this technique. There is a tangible enthusiasm amongst doctors for technology and anaesthesiologists are often ridiculed for their obsession with the latest electronic devices. The three areas of obsession with anaesthesiologists are typically technological devices (normally made by a company named after a fruit also implicated in poisoning Snow White), coffee (our anaesthetic department has a coffee machine worthy of a professional barista) and cycling, triathlons or running marathons in various cities around the world.

Local anaesthetic can be injected either at the level of a peripheral nerve near the tissue damage (as described above) or at their origin from the spinal cord. Many patients who have knee replacements have a spinal anaesthetic, a process in which a needle is inserted into the area where the cerebrospinal fluid circulates and through which small amounts of local anaesthetic are injected. This effectively numbs all the nerves that provide sensation to the legs, rendering the patient numb from the waist down and therefore able to be awake whilst the knee is being replaced – although they might be given some sedation, mainly to avoid the disturbing stream of consciousness which can emanate from some orthopaedic surgeons. This technique can probably be safely practised for operations up to and including a hernia operation done just to the right or left of the belly button, and even for Caesarean sections. The problem is that the higher the local anaesthetic spreads the more likely the patient is to stop breathing. There is therefore a fine line between injecting the local anaesthetic in a great enough quantity to block the relevant nerves for the area being operated on and injecting so much that the patient suffocates.

The spine is not straight but has a concave curve in the lumbar region just above your bum, then is straighter in your middle spine (called the thoracic spine) before having a concave curve in your neck. The trick is to put the local anaesthetic in below the level where the spinal cord ends, usually taken as a point below a line drawn between the tops of your hips. As I'm sure you can imagine, this is a variable target depending on your body type, and sticking a needle right into the spinal cord is never a good idea. The nerves in the cord all run very closely together and with one needle track you can injure the nerves that come from multiple areas of the body.

An alternative to inserting a needle into the fluid-filled space around the spinal cord is to try to find the space that lies between the last ligament of the spinal bones and the lining of the spinal cord, known as the epidural space. This is what we call a potential space because the two layers are separated by dilated veins, and therefore must be accessed via a loss of resistance technique. A needle is inserted into the last ligament layer between two adjacent vertebrae and then a syringe filled either with air or saltwater is attached. When you get to the potential space your syringe plunger suddenly gives way; this is called loss of resistance. Too far and you make a giant hole in the lining surrounding the spinal cord, causing the cerebrospinal fluid to leak and giving the patient a massive headache; not far enough and you are unable to thread the catheter into the space and the local anaesthetic therefore doesn't bathe the nerves as they leave the spinal cord. This technique is relatively easy to do in the bottom region of the spine – unless the reason you're doing it is to ease the pain of labour, in which case it's a bit like trying to sail through the Northwest Passage in a dinghy. The challenge when you try to insert the epidural higher up, at the level of the bottom of the shoulder blades, for operations where the incision will be higher than the belly button is that the two adjacent vertebral bodies are packed tightly on top of one another, virtually obliterating the space that your needle needs to enter, and as pain consultants we are sometimes asked by our anaesthesiologist colleagues to use an X-ray machine to guide the epidural needle into place. Epidurals for pain relief in surgeries such as cutting out a cancer in the food pipe can influence whether you live or die, but for other surgeries a careful assessment is made to establish whether the risks of the epidural, which as mentioned can include permanent nerve damage, are justified. Sometimes epidural catheters fall out and they can become infected, resulting in an abscess around the spinal cord which can, on rare occasions, lead to paralysis.

Another anaesthetic-based drug which is sometimes used to manage chronic pain and pain in the post-operative setting is ketamine. It is a phencyclidine derivative – basically PCP. It was developed in 1962 and used extensively in the Vietnam War as an anaesthetic agent because in the middle of a paddy field you can't intubate the airway to help an injured soldier to breathe, but ketamine, whilst rendering you insensate, does not disturb your ability to protect your breathing passage. There is therefore no risk of you aspirating your stomach contents whilst unconscious. Ketamine is often used now in trauma because it does not cause massive drops in blood pressure like other anaesthetic agents such as propofol. It produces what is called dissociative anaesthesia, where you are unresponsive to pain but completely aware of your surroundings – essentially you enter a trance-like state. We also use it in children for painful procedures; the drug can cause nightmares, which we try to prevent by giving diazepam concurrently, but the risk of a nightmare is more tolerable than giving them drugs that will turn them blue when they stop breathing. Ketamine is also used to medicate horses and recreationally as a drug of abuse.

We use ketamine in the perioperative setting because it blocks receptors at the spinal cord level which are involved in amplifying pain in people who have long-standing pain or where the operation involves such a big incision that it is likely to produce a massive response in the pain alarm system. We give it as an infusion intra-operatively and then it is continued post-operatively to try to reduce the amount of opioid medication that the patient needs to take. As with most anaesthetics, it is really a short-term solution, and long-term use of ketamine damages the brain and bladder, turning the latter into a small, irritable and painful organ.

*

Local anaesthetic blocks are a triumph when the patient is pain-free in the recovery room, or despite having serious heart or lung disease is able to have complex shoulder surgery without general anaesthesia. Unfortunately, the local anaesthetic tends to wear off in the middle of the night and the patient is then left in agony unless it is given through a continuous infusion. Post-operative pain management is therefore complex and fraught with difficulties.

Managing perioperative pain went through a revolution in the nineties when it became clear that we were failing to implement policies to treat post-operative pain in a consistent way. We began to realize that untreated pain has significant effects on the outcome of surgery. Being in pain results in a physiological response; for example, it can cause an increase in heart rate which can cause a heart attack. Or if you have had a big cut in your abdomen, pain might prevent you from breathing deeply because with every breath the pain alarm becomes louder – and so you take shallow breaths, resulting in the bottoms of the lungs collapsing and filling with fluid which then becomes colonized with bacteria. You develop pneumonia and then potentially respiratory failure. Similarly, when you are in pain you are unlikely to want to move, but staying bed-bound causes blood to pool in your legs. When this happens, clots form and bits of clot can break off and travel like missiles to your heart, blocking the outflow of blood. This is called a pulmonary embolism and can result in death when the embolus is large. In these circumstances the clot will resemble a horse's saddle because of the shape it forms in the part of the blood vessel that it lodges in. Usually the clot will break off when the patient first gets up to go to the toilet and bears down. This is therefore often the cause of an instantaneous and undignified end.

As well as altering a patient's behaviour, pain also activates hormones and chemicals which affect the body's ability to heal. We naturally secrete cortisol when we are stressed, a hormone which breaks down protein to make sugar available for muscles to use as energy fuelling flight from our plight. Untreated pain results in an increase in this hormone with the effect that it begins to break down muscle, leading to loss of muscle mass which affects the power of breathing and results in delayed wound healing. This can have catastrophic effects, for example if a surgeon has tried to join two segments of the bowel after excising a cancer, then the delay in healing and potential breakdown of the join can lead to a leak. Leaking fluid inside the abdomen causes inflammation, sepsis and potentially death.

In the nineties and noughties many professional healthcare bodies representing surgeons and anaesthesiologists encouraged hospitals to provide specialist acute pain services. Pain was labelled 'the fifth vital sign' and aggressive pain management was considered both clinically important and a fundamental human right. Perhaps, in retrospect, the zealous pursuit of this goal and linking pain relief to hospital quality outcome measures contributed to the opioid epidemic, which we will come on to in more detail in the next chapter.

The hospital I work at has a large acute pain service consisting of specialist nurses led by a nurse consultant. The pain consultants play a role in managing the more complex cases and are responsible, together with the nurses, for monitoring and implementing policies to make sure that every patient has adequate pain relief and that the latest advances in pain management are implemented in a systematic way. The surgical patient population is growing progressively older, meaning that physiological tolerance to injury is lower and surgeries are more complex, and the more complex the surgery, the more complex the perioperative pain management requirements. Good pain management requires pain-relieving medication protocols that can be consistently prescribed for standard types of operations, whilst bearing in mind potential side effects.

The main aim in perioperative pain medicine these days is enhanced recovery. We used to get people to lie down for ages until they felt better following surgery, but the philosophy of post-operative care now is to get people up and about as soon as possible. Patients who have had major bowel surgery, for example, are up on the first day and the aim of their pain management is to provide good pain relief without constipating the patient up to their eyeballs, which would potentially affect the joining of the bowel segments and suppress the immune system. As discussed above, getting up and about also reduces the risk of developing chest infections and deep vein thrombosis and promotes wound healing, but this can only be accomplished if the blaring pain alarm system is managed effectively.

Pain assessment is fundamental to being able to treat the experience. The Dutch have a saying: you can't manage what you don't measure. As part of their preceptorship courses, newly qualified nurses are therefore trained by the specialist pain nurses in the assessment of pain in order to understand the phenomenon as a complex experience influenced by that individual's unique psychological and social context. The basic principle, therefore, in the medication management of perioperative pain or pain due to trauma is that of a multimodal approach (targeting the different parts of the biological pain alarm system – the nociceptor, spinal cord and brain) supported by an infrastructure to deliver and audit pain management; this usually comes under the auspices of a specialist pain service. The aim is to try to target the different parts of the pain alarm system in order to modify the information received by the individual's brain.

In a healthcare system that is largely biomedical we resort to medications to try to achieve this aim. The evidence base for modulating pain pathways using education and psychological techniques is less well developed, and whilst there is very little money in marketing a behavioural therapy, there is a lot to be gained from developing and selling medication. In the nineties and noughties, opiates were aggressively developed and marketed, with companies generating potent synthetic opioids as well as novel delivery systems (including fentanyl lollipops and nasal sprays) and unfortunately the ubiquitous and sometimes indiscriminate use of opioids led to an undetected epidemic of opioid misuse which is now coming to light.

As part of a multimodal pain-relief strategy we give patients anti-inflammatory medications. We have been using anti-inflammatories in medicine for millennia; the anti-inflammatory agent salicin, the precursor to aspirin, is naturally occurring in willow bark and was known as far back as Hippocrates to be effective for the treatment of fevers. The first anti-inflammatory medication was synthesized by the Bayer pharmaceutical company in 1897, but the mechanism of anti-inflammatory drugs was only elucidated in the 1970s which led to the development of newer agents. Before this mechanism action was fully understood we were already marketing anti-inflammatories that had been developed without the necessary degree of understanding, and many of these drugs are still used today. Examples of these are ibuprofen (the patent for which was filed in 1961) and diclofenac (patented in 1965), which act by blocking prostaglandins from attaching and triggering nociceptors. However, if trialled today, many of these drugs would probably never get past an ethics committee or be given a license for use, given their potential for catastrophic complications in the form of stomach haemorrhage or kidney failure. Even ibuprofen, a common over-the-counter drug available in pharmacies and supermarkets, can cause indigestion, stomach ulcers and, in some individuals, heart and kidney failure.

In an attempt to design safer forms of anti-inflammatory medications, drugs were produced which only acted on the specific enzyme involved in producing the inflammatory chemical which triggers nociceptors and therefore produces pain, but we then found out that if you take these medications long term you have an increased risk of heart attacks and strokes. Anti-inflammatory medications are difficult to give to patients who haven't eaten because blocking the prostaglandins generally stops their protective function in the lining of the stomach, allowing acid to potentially eat through the stomach lining causing an ulcer with resultant bleeding or a hole in the intestine. They are also probably only safe to give for five to seven days after an operation.

If you can't anticipate how much blood loss the patient will suffer in surgery, then giving anti-inflammatories at the beginning of the operation is hazardous because you might further compromise their kidneys. Anti-inflammatory medications also affect the stickiness of platelets which are necessary for clotting and therefore they pose a risk for increased bleeding. Brain operations, for example, are problematic in terms of prescribing anti-inflammatory painkillers because if the patient does bleed it will be into a fixed box containing the brain and the increased blood will crush the brain tissue. Orthopaedic surgeons also don't like them because they believe that anti-inflammatories negatively influence how quickly bones heal. The balance of evidence from experiments on animals suggests that prostaglandins favour bone formation. Non-steroidal anti-inflammatory drugs, or NSAIDs, might be expected to inhibit bone formation because they inhibit prostaglandin formation. Experimental work in animals seems, at best, to demonstrate that the impact of NSAIDs on bone healing after a fracture or operation is uncertain. The evidence is contradictory, there are issues over drug dose and duration, and there is little evidence from clinical practice to support extrapolation to humans.

Trying to block the chemicals that are released when the body is damaged is therefore challenging, and the story of medication for pain is beset with our inability to be precise in terms of blocking harm-sensing information. If in the future we could stop these chemicals from attaching to pain receptors and thereby triggering the electrical signal that the brain interprets as pain, we would not experience pain after surgery – but we are not there yet.

Paracetamol is an oddity as a pain-relieving medication – widely used but, again, poorly understood. Paracetamol is a fever-lowering drug primarily and a very mild painkiller which we think works on cannabinoid receptors (receptors involved in mood, appetite, pain and memory, which are widely found in the body), or possibly on a mystery enzyme, but the truth is that we don't really know how it works. It was accidentally discovered when looking for a cure for intestinal worms. The story goes that two researchers were using naphthalene (a hydrocarbon found in plasterboard, lead batteries, dyes and rubber) as a treatment for killing gut parasites when a pharmacist accidentally delivered a different chemical to them. When they used this chemical in their experiments, they found that it didn't kill the parasites but did lower fevers. The serendipitous mistake by the pharmacist was uncovered and the researchers produced a drug called Antifebrin (from the word 'febrile' meaning fever). Their research stimulated an interest in looking at this class of chemicals further and acetaminophen (paracetamol) was discovered. The drug that was formulated lacked purity, however, and therefore individuals taking the early drug experienced unpleasant side effects such as nausea and headaches.

It wasn't until the 1940s that the metabolism of the toxic metabolites was separated from the positive effects of paracetamol. The drug Trigesic, which was a mixture of aspirin, caffeine and paracetamol, was first marketed in the US in 1950, but unfortunately three patients developed death of all their blood cells which was thought to be related to the paracetamol. In the UK paracetamol was produced as a pure formulation and marketed as Panadol, with the first scientific study concluding that it was not particularly effective as a painkiller compared with codeine. Slowly, however, paracetamol was combined with other medications, increasing its effectiveness as a pain-killer and reducing the side effects, and as the use of aspirin declined as an over-the-counter analgesic, paracetamol increased. Today, paracetamol (marketed as 'Paracetamol – the GP's choice') remains the first-line agent for many people who suffer with aches and pains and headaches or fever, despite only having a modest effect on the former. The story of paracetamol highlights the development of a drug not from first principles of understanding pain or its mechanisms, but from finding an effect and then trying to establish safe use.

The main class of drug that we use to reduce and confuse the messages of harm sent to the brain are opioids, medications that bind to opioid receptors which are present in the body. Opiates have been used since the time of the Ancient Greeks, mainly to treat diarrhoea, insomnia and pain. There are opioids that are naturally produced in the body (endorphins and enkephalins) which attach to these receptors. Opioids either come from the poppy (known as opiates), such as morphine, or are man-made. We used to think that all we were doing in a very benign fashion with the opioids was hyperpolarizing the nerves. This involves making the nerves less excitable by reducing the ability of sodium and potassium ions to flow into and out of the cell. The cells are made more negatively charged and therefore cannot fire off an electrical signal – they become lethargic and depressed. The amount and nature of the transmitted information is thus altered in the spinal cord and consequently by the brain cells receiving the information.

We have always been aware that the reason why opioids are abused is that they affect multiple pathways in the brain, producing changes in mood and motivation. The perceived pain-relieving effect of opioids is now thought to be due to its effect on the emotional component and the individual's reaction to pain, blunting your ability to actively manage or think about the sensations you are experiencing, rather than by blocking nerves or reducing inflammation. Opioids affect how you feel about your pain and your life in general, stifling emotional responsiveness. My patients who have chronic pain and have had the opportunity to reflect on their relationship with opioids, often say to me that when they take their opioids they still have pain, they just don't care as much about it. There are patients who like this effect, and they may be at risk for addiction. And so the theme of empirically using a substance which has effects that we don't really understand continues. Fundamentally this problem arises because we don't really understand pain to a sufficient degree to design drugs that are specific, and because we are using a medication to treat an experience.

*

I spend approximately 20 per cent of my working life managing people with complex pain problems on the wards – either individuals who are struggling with their pain management following surgery or individuals with chronic pain who have been admitted to hospital with a flare-up of their pain. I usually start my ward round at about eight o'clock in the morning, at which point I receive a sheaf of referral forms – and to say that there is a paucity of detail included about the patient would be generous. The referral, which generally appears to be inspired by the admonition of Polonius to Laertes that 'brevity is the soul of wit', usually pithily states: *This patient has had pain for a long time. They have had an operation. Please see with regards to pain management.*

Fortunately, in our hospital we have an extremely robust electronic patient record system and if the patient has been seen by anyone in the hospital before then their outpatient letters will be on the system. One of my first actions is to see whether the person has 'form'. The outpatient letters will detail in coded language the hidden psychosocial distress associated with a long-standing pain condition and the journey that has led them to have an operation which had a very low probability of success. Knowing the patient before you even enter the arena is fundamental to trying to establish the basis for a relationship, the aim of which is to get the patient up, moving, understanding their pain, reducing their distress and reducing their reliance on opiates.

For the average patient the acute severe pain following any surgery usually reduces to manageable levels reasonably quickly. By three weeks following surgery most people only need recourse to over-the-counter pain relief. But what about those who don't take this path? The challenge that we face as anaesthesiologists and consultants working in pain management is where surgery or trauma occurs in an individual where the pain alarm system is already dysfunctional – the person who has established chronic pain (see Chapter Five: Pain with no injury). Particular care needs to be taken with these individuals, as well as those patients who are having surgery that is so destructive – in terms of the amount of tissue that is damaged and the body cavities that are injured – that it causes a massive disruption in the patient's normal physiology and prolonged hyperactivation of the pain alarm, potentially leading to the development of chronic pain. These patients require an augmented approach and additional drugs, together with the more usual opiates, local anaesthetics, paracetamol and anti-inflammatories, are used.

The drugs that we employ in the treatment of complex persistent pain conditions aim to modify the dysfunctional pain alarm system – turning it down, muffling it without suffocating the patient in the process. We also borrow drugs from other disciplines, which attempt to make nerves behave or change brain chemicals, where we have found that there is crossover between dysfunction of the pain alarm system and other conditions. But our understanding of the molecular mechanisms of pain is limited and the medications we borrow from other disciplines have simply been serendipitously discovered to distract the nervous system, rather than being focused on a specific target.

One example of this is the use of antidepressants to manage chronic pain. The original drug used in this regard is amitriptyline, which is one of the older generations of antidepressants and is no longer in common use because of its high risk of overdose. When I worked in South Africa at a hospital in one of the townships, we used to know which patients had been admitted with amitriptyline overdose due to the 'amitriptyline sign' – black discolouration around the patient's mouth due to the ingestion of activated charcoal which is given to treat the overdose because it binds to the drug, preventing absorption into the bloodstream.

The action of antidepressants on chronic pain is due to the pathways that project from the brain down into the spinal cord and which can reduce the amount of electrical information signalling harm that is reaching the brain – the descending inhibitory pathways we came across in Chapter One. In order to function, these pathways require two chemicals or neurotransmitters called serotonin and noradrenaline. When someone is depressed these neurotransmitters are found to be at low levels and therefore the pharmacological treatment of depression with drugs consists of trying to elevate the levels of these chemicals. Patients who are in pain are often found to be depressed and patients who are depressed are more likely to report persistent pain, presumably based on the common biochemical disturbance in these two conditions. In order to activate the descending inhibitory pathways and reduce a patient's perception of pain, the drug needs to be able to raise both serotonin and noradrenaline and therefore drugs like Prozac don't work for persistent pain, as it only results in an increase in serotonin and not noradrenaline. Not every patient responds to treatment with antidepressants, and I suspect that the neurochemical disturbance in persistent pain is much more complex than we currently appreciate.

The initial studies for these drugs were carried out on patients who suffer with nerve pain from diabetes or from shingles, because these conditions provide large groups of relatively similar chronic pain patients. Unfortunately, these neuropathic-pain drugs (antidepressants and anti-epileptic medications) are only effective in about one in seven people and they cause harm in about one in fourteen people. In addition, they only provide about 30 to 50 per cent pain relief, and so I often wonder how many patients are responding to the treatment and how many patients are merely recording a placebo response because something is being given to them, and in fact they are activating their own descending inhibitory pathways merely through the act of being looked after.

The newer antidepressant drugs that we use in pain relief include duloxetine, which started its life as a treatment for incontinence, was then used to treat depression and is now used to treat neuropathic pain, particularly diabetic peripheral neuropathy; this is now a global epidemic as more patients develop diabetes and suffer from the complications that come with this disease. This particular complication is due to the fact that diabetes results in high blood sugar levels which damage the small blood vessels providing nerves with oxygen – the nerves are then damaged and their electrical activity becomes disordered, causing burning, numbness and tingling sensations.

The difficulty when you tell somebody that you are going to give them an antidepressant to help manage their pain is that you reinforce their belief that you consider the pain to be 'all in their head' and imagined, because you have not been able to identify a lesion or area of physical damage. Patients can therefore either get immediately very angry with you, or completely ignore your advice to take the medication.

We also use drugs such as gabapentin and pregabalin to treat pain, borrowed from the world of epilepsy. As with antidepressants, there is considerable crossover in the biochemical disturbances that cause both epilepsy and chronic pain. In neuropathic pain the disturbance is that of the orderly arrangement of channels within a nerve. When you damage a nerve in this way it expresses sodium channels in a haphazard fashion, resulting in the firing of the nerve in a spontaneous and unprovoked manner. The patient feels burning, tingling, stinging and numbness. In epilepsy the aberrant function of nerves may result in seizures or vacant episodes. Gabapentin was named because it was thought to work on the GABA receptor, which is an inhibitory receptor, but it is now believed that it influences calcium channels. Calcium is important for the release of chemicals that cause nerve excitation, and blocking calcium channels in the spinal cord inhibits the release of the excitatory neurotransmitter glutamate. The hyperexcitable nerves of the dysfunctional pain alarm system are therefore tamed to a degree.

Gabapentin has a number needed to treat (NNT) of seven, which means that approximately one person out of seven who you treat with this medication for nerve pain will have approximately 50 per cent pain relief. The NNT is used to indicate the effectiveness of a healthcare intervention. We also talk about numbers needed to harm (NNH), which is the number of people you must give the medication to for one person to develop a significant side effect. The higher the NNH the better the drug. The numbers needed to treat are not good with gabapentin, nor with pregabalin, its more expensive cousin. These drugs have been heavily marketed and sold and we are now in a situation where they are used ubiquitously to treat any pain that goes on for longer than the doctor feels is appropriate. So instead of just being used for chronic nerve pain they are often prescribed for all forms of chronic pain and in the perioperative setting. The effect of these drugs on the patient, however, is to make them foggy and unable to focus and it often makes them feel worse – the taming of the pain alarm also suffocates the patient. Falling over, confusion and sleepiness may result from the use of these nerve-modifying drugs.

Unfortunately, gabapentin and pregabalin have now, like ketamine, found a role as drugs of abuse. I am told these drugs have become very popular in prisons because they facilitate the high from other medications. There is now an awakening that we have flooded the market with these anti-epileptic medications but have not been mindful to monitor their untoward effects and their lack of efficacy. But it is always easier to prescribe somebody a drug – and then walk away. With increasing desperation, we continue to borrow drugs from more and more exotic sources for the management of persistent pain.

Doctors are very good at finding, usually accidentally, pharmacological solutions to complex problems. There is an aphorism that for every complex problem there is a solution which is clear, simple and wrong. Sometimes it is out of desperation in the post-operative setting, where we are managing patients either with difficult to treat acute pain or acute-on-chronic pain, that we prescribe antidepressants and anti-epileptic medication. The prescribing of a drug is often to manage the distress of the prescriber, to alleviate the feelings of helplessness induced in them by the patient, rather than because there is evidence that the drug will be effective in treating the pain. What all these drugs *will* affect, however, are the patient's emotions and thinking – perhaps all we do initially is to provide the patient with a chemical straitjacket.

I often stop medications like gabapentin and antidepressants when they are inappropriately started in the perioperative setting. What prescribers have often failed to tell the patient, or the ward staff, is that these medications take approximately six weeks to reach their maximum efficacy.

The guidance for neuropathic pain is to start patients on either an antidepressant or an anti-epileptic and then after six weeks combine the two. Unfortunately, patients are never told how much pain relief they are supposed to get from these medications and there must be millions and millions of tablets of gabapentin out there which are unused because patients have not been told that for the drug to be effective they have to gradually increase the medication until they experience side effects or reach the maximum allowed dose, and they have not been told that, ultimately, the aim is not complete pain relief. When they then don't get complete pain relief, they tell you that the medication hasn't worked.

*

We don't really understand pain as an experience. Much of its pathways and receptors and its uniqueness in individuals remains a mystery. Because of this, the drugs we use are unrefined and unfocused and as a result often produce unwanted side effects. Despite our lack of understanding, we have created a medical industrial complex which sells the idea that most things can be cured with medication, from your irritable bowel to your depression. The same is true of pain. There is no marketing strategy for the use of mindfulness or meditation to facilitate pain relief or in the management of preoperative anxiety, even though these may be far more effective remedies than the next poorly understood drug. We are also too reliant on operative interventions, destroying tissues in order to somehow produce functional changes that will hopefully improve pain, despite the fact that we understand pain to be complex and know those functional changes have nothing to do with the outcome for the patient. There is very good evidence, for example, that at least 56 per cent of people who have had a technically successful knee replacement continue to experience moderate to severe pain following the surgery. There is as much evidence for the efficacy of conservative treatments that rely on behavioural change such as weight loss and exercise to strengthen quadriceps muscles. But the reality is that most patients prefer to take their chance on the surgery rather than change their behaviour and lifestyle.

Medicating pain throughout the surgical process is important but it is not the whole picture, and several of the medications we use are flawed and dangerous. We often collude with patients in terms of the success of pharmacological management of chronic pain and acute pain. As doctors, we see patients on an irregular basis in the chronic pain setting and so prescribing a medication is an easy undertaking. What we don't see is the gradual decline from a cognitive point of view due to the medication; we don't see the patient falling over and fracturing their hip and coming into hospital and getting pneumonia and dying. We acknowledge the hip fracture and the pneumonia but what we don't acknowledge is the high-dose opioid that made them fall over in the first place. Until now...

The line between pleasure and pain – opioids and addiction

'Among the remedies which it has pleased Almighty God to give to man to relieve his sufferings, none is so universal and so efficacious as opium.'

Thomas Sydenham (the 'father of English medicine')

I started to take codeine and paracetamol. At first it was only once or twice a day, but as the back pain got worse and I struggled to do things on a day-to-day basis and I became more miserable and worried, I found myself taking it every three to four hours – it made me feel better. There were times when the pain became worse and I would not be able to get out of bed and when I went to my GP, he gave me tramadol and he also started me on fast-acting liquid morphine. He told me the medication would help but it didn't, and I went back to him confused about whether to take the codeine, the tramadol or the morphine. The morphine seemed to help the most. It made me feel spaced out during the day though. I tried some injections into my spine, but the back pain never stopped. I started to have the morphine every four to six hours. At first, I used a spoon but eventually I started to just drink it straight from the bottle.

As the years went by, I continued to take the morphine, drinking straight from the bottle; I felt better, less weary and depressed when I took it – at least for a while. I also started to shake if I ran out of morphine. I started to sleep in the middle of the day to help with the pain. The pain clinic told me that I was taking too much morphine and said that they wanted to put me on a patch. I tried the patch, but it didn't help. I continued to take the morphine out of the bottle. I felt my world getting smaller and smaller – just me and my morphine. My GP then started me on long-acting morphine tablets. I didn't find this very helpful and continued to take the liquid morphine.

The pain clinic tried to help by giving me exercises to do and teaching me how to cope with the pain. I still had the pain though and so I asked my GP to increase the long-acting morphine because I was taking more and more of the liquid morphine. Six years after I started taking codeine I was now taking 20 mg of long-acting morphine twice a day and using the liquid morphine every four hours. Nobody could tell me what was wrong with my back and why I had pain. My GP then increased my long-acting morphine to 30 mg. He also tried me on another medication, an antidepressant and anti-epileptic as well as patches of local anaesthetic, but nothing helped.

Eventually I was taking 100 mg of the long-acting morphine and 80 mg of the liquid morphine every day. My GP tried another patch, which he said was equal to about 400 to 600 mg of morphine a day. The patch couldn't stay stuck to my skin, so he switched me back to the liquid morphine. I noticed that my teeth started to rot. I think it was because of the sugar in the liquid morphine. I was using a litre bottle of morphine which would last me about a week or two – sometimes less.

The morphine never helped with my pain. I still had the pain, but I found that I didn't really care about the fact that I had pain. I would be able to sit quietly in the corner and just feel less bad about having pain. The long-acting morphine didn't really help. I suppose it was there in the background doing something, but I never really found that it made me feel as if I could do more things around the house. The liquid morphine was much better and gave me the space to feel a bit less unhappy. It would only last a short period of time and whenever I was really unhappy or distressed, I would take a swig from the bottle. This made me feel a little bit better. The morphine made me constipated, but I used to take laxatives. Sometimes I would have to take the stool out of my bottom with my finger. I never felt particularly well when I was on the morphine, but I felt worse when I wasn't taking it.

The above testimony came from a patient called Diane, who shared this story with me about her relationship with morphine. (We will hear more from Diane in Chapter Six.) Unfortunately, Diane is not alone in her struggle with morphine dependency.

*

Human beings have a long and complex history with opium which dates back to around 5000 BC. Whilst much of its history is medical, opium has also been used recreationally for centuries and Samuel Taylor Coleridge is thought to have composed the poem 'Kubla Khan' as a reflection on his experience with opium. Opium is derived from the opium poppy (*Papaver somniferum*) and is contained within the dried latex obtained from this plant, 12 per cent of which is made up of morphine which can be processed to produce heroin. The latex also contains codeine and thebaine which form the basis of the production of semi-synthetic opioids such as oxycodone and hydromorphone.

Opium was widely cultivated in the ancient world. The Sumerians grew opium poppies as early as 3400 BC and called it the 'joy plant'. The Egyptians cultivated opium in around 1300 BC in the ancient city of Thebes, whose ruins are located in Luxor, which is why the active compound in opium is named thebaine. The Ancient Egyptians restricted the use of opium to priests, who were the gatekeepers of healing and death. Their use of opium was medicinal, and the Ebers Papyrus (*c.*1550 BC), one of the oldest medical papyri discovered, includes a description of opium as a remedy to prevent excessive crying in children, for treating breast infections and for reducing pain during surgical procedures.

The Ancient Greek and Roman civilizations also cultivated the plants, and culling knives used to harvest opium have been found in Cyprus thought to date back to 1100 BC. The trade in opium was widespread in the areas surrounding the Mediterranean Sea, where the oldest seeds from the poppy plant have been found. Hippocrates denounced the magical properties associated with opium but recognized its usefulness for treating pain and disease, for inducing sleep and even for euthanasia. There is evidence that the Greeks used opium in a variety of forms, including inhaling it as a vapour and using it as a suppository. Homer writes in *The Odyssey* that Polydamna, wife of the Egyptian king Thonis, gave Helena, the daughter of Zeus, the mysterious drug nepenthes, which could be slipped into wine and had the power to banish all painful memories. Menelaus and his companions are given nepenthes to forget the horrors of the Trojan War, when these painful memories are recalled by the arrival at court of Telemachus, the son of Odysseus who fought alongside Menelaus. Homer says that nepenthes was grown in the Egyptian fields and the word nepenthes can mean 'no grief' or 'no sorrow' as well as 'no pain', 'painless' or 'cancelling all pain' – it seems likely that the drug being referred to here is some form of opium. Opium was also used as a constituent of the hemlock cup used by the Greeks to ensure a painless death, and the description by Plato of the death of Socrates is consistent with the notion that the fatal drink contained opium.

Whilst the use of intoxicating substances was banned in Islam there is evidence that the use of opium was common in the places conquered by Muslims between 600 and 1500

AD, particularly Turkey where it was drunk as part of a black tea. Arab traders introduced opium to China during the Tang Dynasty (618–907 AD) and to India in roughly 700 AD, and the drug was used by Persian physicians to facilitate anaesthesia for surgical procedures. Persian physicians also recommended opium for the management of melancholy and it was used as an everyday remedy for a variety of aches and ailments in the absence of access to a physician. The effect of opium at the time of the Persians was already known to include pain relief, suppression of coughing, effects on the mind and inhibition of the ability to breathe, as well as disturbance of sexual function.

Opium arrived in Western Europe with soldiers returning from the Crusades between the eleventh and thirteenth centuries but was a taboo subject because in the eyes of the Inquisition anything from the East was from the devil and so was lost to medicine in Europe for more than 200 years. The Swiss physician, astrologer and chemist Paracelsus (or Philippus Aureolus Theophrastus Bombastus von Hohenheim to give him his full birth name), who established the role of chemistry in medicine, encountered opium on his travels in the Middle East in the early sixteenth century. Paracelsus held the view that a doctor must be well-travelled, that knowledge is experience, and is quoted as saying that 'a doctor must seek out old wives, gypsies, sorcerers, wandering tribes, old robbers, and such outlaws and take lessons from them'. He eventually returned to Europe and introduced opium into Western medicine. He is credited with the invention of the drug laudanum, meaning 'worthy of praise', which consisted of opium mixed with amber, crushed pearls, musk and other substances including saffron.

Laudanum remained relatively unknown until an English physician, Thomas Sydenham, proposed his own proprietary formulation in the seventeenth century, and recommended its use for a variety of ailments. In a world of appalling living conditions where individuals were beset with diarrhoea due to cholera, with persistent coughs and with various other pains, an opiate-based medicine represented a panacea, and Sydenham's laudanum retained its popularity well into the eighteenth century. Opium was an effective treatment for cholera and diarrhoea because it causes constipation, and was also used for joint pain and difficulty with sleeping. The only alternatives to laudanum from a medical point of view at this time were poisonous substances such as arsenic, mercury or drugs designed to induce vomiting.

Where there was psychological disequilibrium, opium also found its place. The effects of opioids in the form of alleviating anxiety and increasing dopamine levels with consequent production of euphoria resulted in its popularity amongst physicians who even recommended it for people without any maladies in order to equilibrate the internal environment of the body. The sedative effects of opiates were used to treat patients with psychosis throughout the eighteenth century, and administering opioids was considered a more humane treatment than the restraint methods that until then had been the predominant form of psychiatric treatment based on the idea that people with mental health problems were insensitive animals. In the US, opioid prescription further increased in the nineteenth century because it was ubiquitously given to women suffering from complaints that were attributed to their gender and which included menstrual pain and hysteria.

*

Opium also played a major political and economic role in the history of China. One of the earliest records of opium use in China dates back to 1483, in which it is described as aiding masculinity and enhancing the art of sex through delayed ejaculation. The introduction of tobacco smoking to China by the Portuguese in the 1500s is perhaps responsible for the use of opium becoming more extensive, because opium was then mixed with tobacco, transforming the use of opium from an indulgence of the elite to a widespread phenomenon. It was feared by the ruling elite that groups of opium smokers congregating in the southern provinces of China were plotting against the Emperor. Given the calming effect of opiates, this fear of a revolutionary predisposition is likely to have been unfounded. The social ills caused by opium as well as the authorities' fear of these groups of 'opium-eaters' led to decrees banning the use of the drug. The first opium ban and prohibition began in 1729 in China, and it was completely banned from 1799 until 1860.

By the eighteenth century China was known as the silver graveyard of the world because it had a positive trade balance, particularly with England. We wanted tea, silk and porcelain – but mainly tea – and in return we paid in silver. In order to balance this deficit, the English traded opium illegally to the Chinese in order to support the British addiction to tea. In 1839 the First Opium War was triggered when the Chinese commissioner destroyed 20,000 chests of opium supplied by the British as payment for tea – burning the drug with fire, salt and lime and flushing it into the sea. The event took place on 3 June, which is still the date commemorated as anti-drug day in China. The British government was not willing to pay for their tea with silver, as opposed to the cheap opium produced in India which formed the usual and unofficial payment, and so began the First Opium War. The Treaty of Nanking was signed consequently when the Chinese were defeated, and as part of the treaty the British were given the barren rock in the ocean which would become Hong Kong.

The Imperial Commissioner of Canton, however, was determined to stamp out the opioid trade and closed Canton off to foreign traders. The ensuing conflict with the British and the French who sought to regain this gateway to China resulted in the Second Opium War, from 1856 to 1860. The Chinese defeat resulted in the forced legalization of the opioid trade, the expansion of trade in cheap labour and exemption of foreign imports from internal trade tariffs. China began massive domestic production of opium; it is estimated that by 1905 approximately 25 per cent of the male Chinese population were regular consumers of opium and by 1906 13.5 million people across the country were consuming 39,000 tons of opium per year. The Second Opium War opened trade to the West as part of the Chinese defeat in this war – five more Chinese ports were opened to direct foreign trade rather than having to engage with the government. It can therefore be argued that opium is the reason why China did not continue to be an isolationist empire retreating behind the Great Wall. It is also easy to understand why today the Chinese might feel aggrieved at being lectured by Western powers about human rights violations and the production and export of Chinese-made fentanyl, a potent synthetic opioid used by anaesthesiologists in hospitals for pain relief after surgery and in a slow-release patch formulation for chronic pain, and which is widely regarded to be fuelling the current opioid crisis in the US.

In the latter part of the nineteenth century, there was widespread movement of Chinese and Indian workers to other parts of the world, particularly the western United States to engage in mining, railroad construction and agriculture. These workers brought with them the habit of opium smoking, and established opium dens called Chinatowns. This was particularly the case with Chinese immigrants moving to the US, and restrictions were soon introduced with regards to who could use opium, for fear that the local populations would become addicted. The Chinese migration in 1849 to San Francisco in California led to the formation of the International Opium Commission, a body designed to instigate the global prohibition of drugs.

*

Opioids refer to naturally occurring and synthetic substances that bind to opioid receptors within the body. Opiates with a 't' are obtained from the opium poppy, *Papaver somniferum*; for example morphine, codeine and thebaine are active compounds derived from the plant. Morphine (named after Morpheus, the Ancient Greek god of dreams) was first synthesized in Germany in 1804 by Friedrich Sertürner and was produced in industrial quantities in Germany in the 1820s. The development of the syringe by Alexander Wood in 1855 resulted in the ability to administer morphine easily and frequently, perhaps contributing inadvertently to the overuse of opiates. The use and administration of opiates were not regulated in the 1800s or early 1900s, prior to the Harrison Narcotics Tax Act of 1914, and individuals could obtain morphine for a variety of ailments. The Sears and Roebuck catalogue for example offered morphine and a syringe for $1.50. Alcohol-based treatments were also widespread – if it made you feel good, it must be good for you seemed to be the prevailing view. 'Headache powders' containing opium were available over the counter and were self-administered without recourse to medical assessment or diagnosis. It wasn't until the mid-nineteenth century that doctors began to realize that the regular use of morphine resulted in negative effects.

Heroin, which is a derivative of morphine, was first chemically synthesized by C. Wright in 1874 and was introduced to the market by the Bayer Company of Germany in 1895 as a less addictive form of morphine, sold under the trademark Heroin as an over-the-counter remedy for cough suppression. The name Heroin was coined based on the German word for 'strong' and 'heroic'. At the time, morphine was a popular recreational drug, and was widely available, given that it found its way into many patented remedies such as Mrs Winslow's Soothing Syrup (morphine and alcohol) recommended for fussy children, and formulations for menstrual cramps, and therefore Bayer wished to find a similar but less addictive alternative – hence the development of Heroin. By the mid-twentieth century heroin became a problem as the recreational drug of choice amongst jazz and rock musicians. It is interesting that human beings don't learn at all, and Purdue Pharma would make the same mistake marketing oxycodone (a synthetic opioid) as a less addictive alternative to morphine some hundred years after Bayer first marketed Heroin.

By 1910 there was an epidemic of heroin use in the US, since working-class Americans had learnt to crush the pills into powder and inhale it to achieve a concentrated euphoria. The Harrison Narcotics Tax Act was passed in 1914 in the US to regulate morphine because of this rising level of addiction to heroin. The anthropologist Michael Agar talks interestingly about heroin being the ideal drug for New York, a city that delivers a constant information overload. He refers to heroin as the audiovisual technology that helps manage that overload by dampening it across the board, allowing you to focus on one small aspect of it, on a scale that the human perceptual equipment was designed to handle. Perhaps this is the reason why chronic pain patients find morphine useful sometimes – it dulls and distracts.

Heroin was eventually banned by the League of Nations in 1925; however, this led to the production of related drugs such as oxymorphone and hydrocodone in massive quantities because of the gap in the market left by abandoning the production of heroin. The Committee on Drug Addiction, formed under the banner of the National Research Council in 1929, supervised research into the morphine molecule in order to find a non-addictive, safe alternative to morphine. As a result of this research several different opiate analgesics were derived, including oxycodone and methadone, but the strong, non-addictive alternative to morphine which the researchers set out to develop has still not been realized.

In the UK, the Department of Health's Rolleston Committee report established guidelines in 1926 for the use and prescription of diamorphine (the chemical compound of which Heroin is a trademarked product), and heroin continues to be widely used in palliative care in the UK today. Some users believe that it causes more euphoria than other kinds of morphine, which may be related to the way it is metabolized to morphine in the body. It is more potent than morphine because it is more fat-soluble and therefore more rapidly absorbed by the brain. Unfortunately, heroin also continues to be a major drug of abuse in the UK.

Shortly after marketing Heroin, Bayer had synthesized aspirin in 1899 and this became an over-the-counter drug worldwide after 1917; for the majority of the global population aspirin became the drug of choice used to treat pain, rather than opiates. For cancer pain, however, opiates remained essential. There was a growing criticism of doctors who withheld morphine from patients suffering with cancer, but these doctors were conflicted between the choice of relieving the individual's pain whilst risking possible addiction. Opiates were therefore withheld until the last few weeks of a patient's life.

Dame Cicely Saunders (1918–2005), regarded as the founder of palliative medicine in the UK and responsible for establishing the first purpose-built hospice in 1967, was a strong proponent of using opiates for cancer pain. She developed the Brompton Cocktail, a mixture of morphine, cocaine and gin, in order to ease the suffering of her patients and improve their deaths. She coined the term 'total pain', which she described as a clinical phenomenon that compounded physical and mental distress with social, spiritual and emotional concerns. Studies done at St Christopher's

Hospice by Robert Twycross demonstrated that morphine was superior to and more efficient than heroin, and reported the absence of tolerance or addiction in cancer patients even with long-term use. In 1982 the World Health Organization (WHO) Cancer Unit convened to produce the WHO Ladder, a set of guidelines for physicians managing cancer pain, recommending that they prescribe analgesics on a regular three-step schedule, and measure and adjust the dosage according to the patient's pain at each of the three steps – starting with anti-inflammatory medications like aspirin, moving on to codeine and finally morphine. Some physicians began to recommend the application of this ladder to patients with chronic non-cancer pain, but there remained concerns with regards to prescribing opiate medications in this situation. If you ask medical students today how to manage any kind of pain their answer will be 'the WHO ladder', so powerfully has this approach been marketed, even though it is rarely appropriate for acute pain and is inappropriate for chronic non-cancer pain.

In 1986 the WHO published its 'Cancer Pain' monograph and the management of cancer pain became a priority in many countries; however, there are still some countries today that suffer from poor management of cancer pain with opioids, due to the pejorative connotations of opioid use. In the 1990s there were several further publications looking at the under-treatment of pain and questions were asked about why opioids were solely reserved for cancer pain and avoided in non-cancer pain states. The work of

Kathleen Foley in the 1970s at Memorial Sloan Kettering Cancer Center in New York was geared towards understanding the use of opioids in cancer pain. Her belief was that the censures against opioids made little sense. She was influenced by the work of her mentor, Raymond Houde, who conducted crossover studies of analgesics in cancer patients showing that morphine was superior to other forms of pain relief. Houde's crossover studies indicated that it was a misconception that morphine-type drugs enslaved, demoralized and led the unwitting patient down the path to addiction. Foley was also influenced by the work of Cicely Saunders and Robert Twycross who were using regular heroin dosages to free patients from what they perceived to be the twenty-four-hour nightmare of constant pain. They viewed the patient's pain as being of greater harm than any potential risk of developing dependency on morphine.

Unfortunately, the push from cancer pain specialists to treat their patients with opioids spilled over into that of chronic non-cancer pain, leading to an indiscriminate and unreflective assessment of the differences between cancer and non-cancer pain. Foley published articles in 1981 and 1986 indicating the low incidence of addictive behaviour in small groups of cancer and non-cancer patients. The first one was published as a one-paragraph letter without detailing any scientific method as to how the conclusions were reached. The authors asserted that there was a 0.03 per cent risk of addiction for patients receiving opioids for acute pain. The other study looked at thirty-eight patients and was a retrospective case review. According to this evidence only two out of the thirty-eight patients with chronic pain developed issues in terms of misuse or abuse when receiving opioids. This inadequate evidence became the scientific basis for a twenty-year campaign for the long-term use of opioids in cases of chronic non-cancer pain, led by Foley and her colleague Russell Portenoy. Dr Portenoy later said in a 2010 videotaped interview, 'I gave innumerable lectures in the late 1980s and 90s about addiction that weren't true', and that it was 'quite scary' to think how the growth in opioid prescribing driven by people like him had contributed to soaring rates of addiction and deaths due to overdose. Portenoy was sponsored by Purdue Pharma and other companies to promote the use of opioids in chronic non-cancer pain but has denied that these financial relationships influenced his views.

Chronic non-malignant pain and cancer pain are both complex biopsychosocial phenomena. The difference between the two is that cancer pain in the palliative care setting has a terminal endpoint with regards to the prescribing of opioids because the patient usually dies and is not trying to hold down a job or look after a family. Interestingly it is now known that high-dose opioids used to treat cancer pain may in fact affect the absolute longevity and quality of life of the individual. This may be because of the immunosuppressive effect of opioids which accelerates the cancer.

Unexplained pain is particularly hard to treat, and in the 1920s these patients were regarded as deluded, malingering or were accused of being drug abusers. Unfortunately, despite what we now know about pain, this is still sometimes the explanation offered to patients who suffer with chronic non-cancer pain. In the 1970s there was increasing criticism of the failure of clinicians to treat patients with adequate doses of opioids and in the 1980s a widespread belief developed that the use of opioids for therapeutic indications rarely resulted in addiction. The evidence base for this assertion were the two small retrospective publications (previously described) by Foley from 1981 and 1986. The use of opioids for chronic non-cancer pain was therefore based on two small studies without any prospective follow-up regarding safety issues or extensive studies randomizing groups of patients with pain conditions and testing whether opiates were of benefit.

In 1995 the American Pain Society launched a campaign labelling pain as the fifth vital sign. The aim of this movement was to encourage the standardized evaluation and treatment of pain symptoms. The Veterans Health Administration lent support to this campaign and in 1999 they too adopted the idea of pain as the fifth vital sign. Further government input emphasized the need for assessment of pain. The change in how opioids were seen in the management of pain was aided by the Drug Enforcement Administration which promised less regulatory scrutiny over doctors who prescribed opioids; these doctors were also promised support by the Federation of State medical boards. Hospitals implemented these new changes and instituted systems for pain assessment. The same revolution in the aggressive management of pain was seen in the UK with the start of inpatient pain services to manage acute pain following the report 'Pain After Surgery' published in 1990, which highlighted the inadequacies of post-operative pain management in UK hospitals. In the US pain management was mandated and if benchmarks around pain assessment were not met then a hospital was likely to be penalized. American hospitals therefore invested heavily in opioid therapy in order to receive better satisfaction ratings amongst their patients.

Pharmaceutical companies also got on board and heavily pushed the use of opioids, aggressively marketing them under the banner of being a humane treatment option. It is calculated that in the last twenty years approximately $8 billion was paid in inducements to physicians to expound on the safety and benefits of opioids in the US. Trainees in pain medicine and other specialties were taught to rely on opioids for pain treatment. Newer formulations such as oxycodone were introduced and were marketed as being opiates with a lower likelihood of abuse. However, oxycodone has been heavily abused – renamed 'hillbilly heroin' in some states in the US. Between 1997 and 2002 oxycodone prescriptions increased from 670,000 to 6.2 million in the US, and overall opioid consumption rose from 46,946 kg in the year 2000 to a peak of 165,525 kg in 2012.

The belief initially was that the rise in opioid consumption did not appear to increase the risks of complications in the perioperative setting. However, concerns soon arose with an almost twofold increase in incidents of over-sedation due to opioids; a link started to be established between overaggressive pain management and this substantial increase in over-sedation associated with fatal respiratory depression. Between 1999 and 2016 opioid sales quadrupled and mortality rates in both men and women as a result of opiate use also quadrupled. Evidence of increasing pain, worsening disability, hormonal problems and increased anxiety and depression have also emerged related to opioid use. Despite this increasing mortality rate and the ubiquitous use of morphine to treat chronic non-cancer pain, there has been no Level I evidence (a randomized control trial choosing a condition and then giving one group the opioid and the other a placebo) evaluating the efficacy or safety of the use of opioids in chronic non-cancer pain in terms of reducing pain and improving function.

During the 1990s the aggressive marketing in America of OxyContin (the brand name of oxycodone) by Purdue Pharma intersected with the trafficking of heroin in cities across the Midwest. OxyContin was marketed as being low risk of addiction because it was a prolonged release formulation – but the situation was a repeat of the crisis a hundred years earlier when Bayer had produced Heroin as a less addictive alternative to morphine, as users soon realized that they could crush or snort the OxyContin in order to still achieve a high. Liberal prescriptions were written by overworked GPs with no access to multidisciplinary pain clinics. Once recognized, the misbranding of OxyContin by Purdue Pharma resulted in them having to pay fines of $634.5 million in 2007. They were accused of intentionally downplaying the risk of addiction posed by OxyContin and misleading physicians and the healthcare industry by overstating the benefits of opioids for chronic pain. Purdue therefore agreed to cut its sales force in half and stop promoting opioids.

When OxyContin became too expensive in the late noughties the use of black tar heroin increased, particularly in middle America. Whilst the US had a long-standing problem with heroin, the increased number of people initially hooked on prescription opioids but who then found them too expensive and therefore switched to heroin exacerbated historical heroin abuse. Over time heroin came to be seen by middle-class Americans and adolescents as well as young adults as being less stigmatized and taboo because of their gateway use of OxyContin. In the last decade, deaths due to drug overdose have increased 137 per cent across America and overdoses involving prescription opioids and heroin have increased by 200 per cent.

We are now in the grip of an opioid epidemic – again.

The epidemic, identified due to the staggering increase in opioid-related deaths in the US, was declared on 16 October 2017 and is considered a public health emergency. In 2016 64,000 people died from drug overdoses and, of those, 42,000 were opioid deaths, representing a 20 per cent increase from

2015. Illegally manufactured fentanyl represents the greatest contribution to this increase. The opioid epidemic has now even reached popular culture. Fictional star of page and screen Jack Reacher has been exposed to the opioid epidemic and David Baldacci has written a novel which depicts opioid misuse in middle America. The BBC has now produced programmes on opioids and their effect on society.

The opioid epidemic demonstrates our destructive tendency to treat a complex experience such as pain with a medication in the absence of a clear understanding of the myriad chemical interactions that underpin this phenomenon. A hammer has been used to crack a nut and, even though sometimes the nut is revealed, it is no longer edible.

But what is the alternative to a biomedical approach spearheaded by doctors armed with medicines, scalpels and needles? In American alone 25 million adults suffer with chronic pain and 23 million with severe recurrent pain; one in seven adults in the UK population are thought to suffer with chronic non-cancer pain. This leads to disability and loss of work productivity as well as compromised quality of health and life. Clearly a solution is needed. Rather than relying on opioids, we need to adopt a biopsychosocial approach to the management of pain, including pain management programmes based on cognitive behavioural therapy, relaxation and coping skills, and even self-hypnosis. Unfortunately, insurers regard this approach as being too costly and the prescribing of an opioid appears, on the surface, to be a much simpler solution.

The International Association for the Study of Pain declared in Montreal in 2010 that the relief of pain and suffering is a moral duty of physicians and that access to adequate pain relief is a fundamental human right – but we have now swung the other way, with pain assessment seen as dangerous because it leads to excessive opioid prescribing. What should be assessed is not the pain score but the impact of pain on function. I would, for example, say to a patient who has fractured ribs that the aim of pain relief is to facilitate deep breathing and coughing to prevent a chest infection, rather than treating a number that has been ascribed to the level of pain.

New standards in pain management now include recommendations relating to psychosocial risk factors that may affect the self-reporting of pain, the setting of realistic goals and developing treatment plans that focus on the ability of a medication to increase physical functioning. The guidance for assessing whether a pain medication should be used, and the outcome measures which are to be assessed, now follow the Initiative on Methods, Measurement and Pain Assessment in Clinical Trials (IMMPACT) recommendations. The effect of the medication should be evaluated in terms of: (1) pain, (2) physical functioning, (3) emotional functioning, (4) participant ratings of improvement and satisfaction with treatment, (5) symptoms and adverse events, and (6) participant disposition (e.g. adherence to the treatment regimen and reasons for premature withdrawal from the trial).

*

Chronic pain is often found to develop in patients who have undergone repeated abdominal operations and episodes of inflammation, resulting in a hyperactive and sensitive pain alarm system. These patients develop what is called visceral neuropathic pain or chronic abdominal pain. The difficulty with pain that comes from an organ as opposed to pain that comes from a muscle or a ligament is that the nerves to an organ are very poorly localized and hitchhike with nerves that go to muscles. If you have ever experienced diarrhoea you will remember and recall the unpleasant colicky sensation from bowels that are behaving abnormally and how the pain seems to be everywhere. The constant pain is accompanied by an inability to eat. Patients who have chronic abdominal pain therefore have a miserable existence, and their distress usually leads to the prescribing of high-dose opioids.

By the time pain specialists such as myself are called to see patients with intestinal failure, the patient is usually already on high-dose opiates and the reason we are asked to see them is to rationalize the use of their opiates, which is like taking a teenager's phone away from them – forever. Often patients have developed certain habits, which might include wanting opiates to be only given by injection, even after they have started to eat and drink again. The explosion in the types of opiates which can be given, and the variety in routes of entry, means that patients who cannot eat and drink are often given these newer formulations such as lollipops, sprays and patches, which can reinforce addiction. Fentanyl lollipops containing high doses of fentanyl which is absorbed through the mouth, and intranasal opiates which can be inhaled, are both routes that favour the development of addiction as they produce rapid and profound effects because of the nature of the absorption.

When we go and see these patients we battle to try to introduce the concept of chronic pain and begin a conversation about the harm that opiates can cause. In somebody who is miserable and who suffers with chronic abdominal pain it is very hard for them to accept that what you are offering is better in the long term than the temporary but immediate escape offered by an opioid. Battles therefore rage around opioid reduction. I sometimes wonder when I go on these wards whether it is not kinder to just allow the patient to have their opiates.

Despite several decades of research into the complexity of pain and how it should be assessed and managed, patients, aided by the medical profession, continue to want a simple pharmaceutical solution to their pain. Concerns around the use of opioids and their lack of efficacy in the management of chronic non-cancer pain, as well as the serious side effects associated with long-term use, have resulted in the search for a different pharmacological agent. These days the most commonly asked question that I hear in the pain clinic is about cannabis oil. Cannabis may now represent a continuation of our ongoing missteps in the management of chronic pain.

The understanding of what goes wrong in the way nerves behave in pain without injury is undeveloped and drug companies therefore do not have a precise target to aim for when trying to develop medicines for pain. Pain, however, is an emotional experience and seeing somebody in pain evokes the desire to rescue, on the part of the healthcare worker as well as that individual's loved ones. This need to alleviate pain in others is what led to the opioid crisis in the first place, when we decided to champion the idea of managing this experience and, through our hubris, felt that we could do so from a medical point of view, ignoring the fact that chronic pain is an experience and needs to be approached from a biopsychosocial point of view.

We have still not learnt our lesson and are now once again approaching the same experience and trying to modify it with another pharmacological agent in the form of cannabis. Industry has got on board and cannabis stocks have soared. So instead of calming down and assessing where this medication fits into the management of specific pain conditions and then carefully conducting randomized controlled trials in order to assess which patients benefit from what dose and what formulation of the drug, we are steaming forwards again. When you take one tool away from doctors, in order to sustain their position as providers of healthcare they move on to another medication that can be controlled and prescribed. There have so far only been twelve randomized controlled trials on cannabis in the last five years and most of these studies have indicated that cannabinoids are not effective in the management of neuropathic pain. There is a real danger that we will supplant one mind-altering substance with another, all because we cannot appreciate that health and well-being is about more than pharmacological agents that can simply be packaged and sold.

Over the years we have used, abused and promoted the use of opium. What is also clear is that whilst opium has been used for pain it is not the predominant narrative in the relationship we have had with the drug. We have used its tranquilizing, constipation-inducing, cognitive and behavioural modification effects far more. It becomes clear that using opium for pain is about managing the behaviour of the sufferer rather than arresting the pain alarm or treating the cause.

Our dysfunctional history with opiates perhaps reflects our struggles with the slings and arrows of life itself. The opioid epidemic and the deaths caused by opiate use have been termed 'deaths of despair', implying that opioid abuse reflects deeper societal issues alongside our complex relationship with understanding pain. Pain may be due to physical injury but the discomfort we feel when we are emotionally distressed is no less unpleasant than a broken bone. When life becomes too much and we feel overwhelmed we may try to cope by pushing these feelings down with alcohol, sugar, opioids and cannabis. These drugs all narrow the way we see the world and cause our brain's ability to perceive the world to shrink, lessening out anxiety and despair.

This relationship that we have had with opiates is a cautionary tale. The fact that physicians working in cancer pain management, who heroically want to save the patient from suffering and are involved in the care of the dying, were able to state with very little supporting evidence that morphine is perfectly safe in managing pain in a non-terminal condition is a worrying example of how a therapy can be introduced despite little evidence for its benefits and centuries of recorded harm. It is extraordinary how the lessons of history have not been heeded with regards to our relationship with opiates. There is so much repetition to be seen in the introduction of the Harrison Narcotics Tax Act in 1914, the Opium Wars and the introduction of Heroin a hundred years ago, reflected more recently in the wars in Afghanistan, the introduction of oxycodone and our current opioid epidemic.

Over a hundred years ago, in the *New York Times* in 1911, the Opium Commissioner Dr Hamilton Wright was quoted as saying:

Of all the nations of the world, the United States consumes the most habit-forming drugs per capita. Opium, the most pernicious drug known to humanity, is surrounded, in this country, with far fewer safeguards than any other nation in Europe fences it with. China now guards it with much greater care than we do; Japan preserves her people from it far more intelligently than we do ours, who can buy it, in almost any form, in every tenth one of our drug stores.

Those who ignore the lessons of history are doomed to repeat its mistakes.

*

When it comes to treating pain, we sway from one end of the spectrum to another like the length of dresses. Skirts get longer, and skirts get shorter with no real rhyme or reason. All the while, those who prescribe opioids probably don't take them, and those who take the opioids are probably never given enough information about the harm they are causing. We would rather provide a single drug – and now cannabis is rearing its head – than admit that people need to understand and learn to manage their pain, and we would rather prescribe a medication than invest in psychology therapies or physiotherapy services.

One of the main functions of the pain clinic I work in is now to help people reduce their opioid use. The conversation with the patient who was prescribed opioids is difficult. How do you have a conversation where you say: well the drug which has been given to you, and which you are now on, and which had no evidence base, is poisoning you. The contract between patient and doctor when starting opioid treatment is not merely writing the prescription but should include documentation of a discussion around the risks and benefits of the therapy – but historically this has not been the case. GPs who have for years prescribed opioids like Smarties are now asking us to position ourselves as an opioid-reduction clinic. And because pain services are under threat because pain injection therapies are being stopped, we have decided that this is probably the way forward.

There may be a role for the use of opioids in chronic pain, but it is not a role that we have studied and therefore we do not have the necessary information to recommend its use. We have evidence regarding the effective use of opioids in the management of acute post-operative pain but increasingly realize that we should be more cautious in their use, monitoring for signs of addiction and limiting the amount that is given to patients.

The reality in medicine is that we act these days as if we've cracked it. We believe that because we are so technologically advanced, and we have these magnificent temples called hospitals, that we have all the answers. The reality is far different, and we therefore swing from one failed pharmacological or surgical therapy to another without appreciating or admitting that the solutions to healthcare problems in the first world are complex. Poor lifestyles cannot be medicated, and wellness cannot be prescribed.

Until patients challenge doctors and engage much more in the decision-making around their situation, we will probably continue in our current vein, and in the next hundred years we will probably swing back to prescribing opioids ubiquitously – or perhaps the new morphine is cannabis.

Pain with no injury

U sually pain goes away, not dramatically, like an unwanted guest leaving your house, but quietly. At the end of its time with you it becomes an itch at the edge of your perception and then eventually it is no longer present at all. The alarm switches off because your body has healed. There are times, however, when despite all the tissues knitting together, pain persists.

Pain is usually perceived in society to be a symptom of injury or harm and the main preoccupation of the doctor is to find out what the cause of the pain is. Doctors often employ an approach to medicine which involves gathering many pieces of information and whittling it down to a single diagnostic label, aiming to reduce the complexity presented by individuals with persistent pain and a multitude of symptoms down to a single point of origin – a pain generator.

But pain is a very complex biological alarm system. It is biologically ancient with pathways that are hardwired into multiple areas of the brain, and it is not as specific a guide to danger as we like to think it is. Dysfunction of the organs, for example, like the heart or the pancreas, results in poorly localized pain to the left arm and the middle of the stomach respectively. The specificity of pain as a symptom is therefore often overestimated. A straightforward diagnosis – a pain generator – cannot always be found. The tools employed by doctors to reach such a diagnosis have traditionally been taking a history of pain (medical students were encouraged to use the mnemonic derived from Socrates when assessing pain: site, onset, character, radiation, associations, time course, exacerbating/relieving factors and severity), the ordering of investigations and performing a clinical examination.

Medical students today, in contrast, are increasingly taught the Calgary Cambridge method of consultation. First the doctor will make every attempt to build rapport by asking open questions and employing active listening techniques, placing the patient at the centre of care. At the same time information will be collected in order to assess both the disturbance in the person's physiology (the disease) as well as an understanding of the psychosocial factors which may impact on the disease. The change in how doctors assess patients is rooted in the understanding that *disease* and *illness* are two very different concepts: disease is what the doctor says that the patient has, and illness is what the patient suffers with. Doctors assess and treat for disease, whilst patients report illness. The disease is determined through a process similar to the old method, by taking a history, performing an examination and ordering investigations in order to narrow down the possibilities with regards to what is different from normal or not functioning properly. The concept of *illness* attempts to understand that disease within the context of the patient, because this has implications in terms of how successfully that condition may be treated. Unfortunately, most doctors still operate a reductionist model and the psychosocial aspect of a patient's health is often ignored.

Lower-back pain, for example, is a universal human affliction and is often attributed to dysfunction of various components of the spine, which is a very complex structure consisting of vertebral bodies stacked one on top of the other. Various tests have been devised by doctors in order to mimic the pain which the patient presents with and therefore identify the pain generator – the source of the problem and the bit of the patient's back that can be fixed with screws and rods, cut out with a scalpel or made numb by burning its nerve supply. This follows the reductionist trap of trying to refine a disease and define a disease process. Unfortunately, the spine is not a structure which is easily defined in such terms and the innervation of the spine is complex; one nerve may in fact give sensation to multiple structures.

Whilst nociception is the detection of harmful stimuli by specialized receptors and nerve endings, and this information that damage has occurred to the body is transmitted to the spinal cord and brain, pain is the way that the individual *perceives* this harmful information. Pain occurs due to the person filtering the information about harm through their past life experiences and current psychological make-up. The information about harm is also filtered through the cultural and social lens of that person, and the presentation to the GP with symptoms of pain will very much depend on the individual's psychosocial context.

Thinking about human beings as being a separate mind and body rather than an integrated entity leads to a poor assessment and insufficient management in healthcare. When the body is seen as a machine and the focus is on looking for a disease, a disruption of bones and ligaments or dysfunction of organs, then the impact of psychological and social factors on both the initial reporting of symptoms and on the subsequent response to treatment is ignored, leading to inadequate management and a lack of progress in terms of improving function.

As we have explored, pain is an abnormal sensation emanating from somebody's body and is interpreted through their own unique experiences and understanding of normal. Pain is the final expression of what the individual understands about their bodies and their tolerance for discomfort. When it comes to perceiving and understanding pain in others, pain is culturally determined: where pain is due to an obvious cause, such as a broken limb or a musculoskeletal strain, then it is relatively easy to understand; where pain occurs insidiously and progressively it is more difficult to understand. We are as a species meaning-makers, and without an understanding of our pain from a doctor we will develop our own narratives rooted within our cultural context. So, what happens when there is pain and illness that has persisted beyond the normal period of healing, but no evidence remains of the initial disease, injury or ongoing tissue damage? At this point, a patient is said to suffer from chronic pain.

Chronic pain is divided into two categories: primary chronic pain syndromes (e.g. fibromyalgia syndrome, complex regional pain syndrome, non-specific lower-back pain) and secondary chronic pain syndromes. Primary chronic pain is defined as pain in one or more anatomical regions that persists or recurs for longer than three months and is associated with significant emotional distress or functional disability (that is to say, it interferes with the activities of daily life and restricts participation in social roles) and that cannot be better accounted for by another (non-primary) chronic pain condition. This is a new definition, which applies to chronic pain syndromes that are best conceived as health conditions in their own right. Secondary chronic pain is persistent pain where the initial cause was as a result of cancer, nerve injury or trauma: the pain, for example, which persists after a whiplash injury has healed is a secondary chronic pain syndrome; pain which persists after an episode of shingles is a secondary chronic neuropathic pain syndrome due to the virus having damaged nerves.

*

I first met Helen on a Saturday. I sometimes run pain clinics on a Saturday when the hospital is quiet, and I feel I have more space to breathe (it also enables me to get out of doing the Saturday cleaning at home). She was very fashionably dressed and was accompanied by her husband. They seemed like a loving and attentive couple – the partner who attends the appointment usually is; sometimes too attentive to be helpful. She had the usual air of reticence that I often see in patients who have been referred to a clinic named after a symptom. Neurosurgical clinic, cardiology clinic, respiratory clinic – these are clinics that inspire confidence of a cure. Not so a pain (management) clinic. Helen had been referred by a neurosurgeon because she had complained of pain in her arms and legs. The neurosurgeon had explained to her that there was no target for an operation on her spine which would cure her pain. She did not receive this information well because she'd had two previous operations on her neck and assumed that the symptoms that she was experiencing were symptomatic of the same problem, and so she could not understand why she was not being offered a third operation (not that the other two operations had resolved her symptoms – I am always amazed and a little bit envious of the faith that people have in surgeons and their scalpels).

Helen was forty-eight and worked as a nurse in an operating theatre, which often involves standing for long periods of time assisting with operations. Often operations will last for three or four hours – scrub nurses have to open up large, heavy trays and keep an eye on the number of swabs used in case one gets left inside the patient, which is easier to do than you might think. Helen had two children in their teens and an older child who has children of his own. She was therefore mother, grandmother, wife and NHS worker. I asked about her pain symptoms and she said that she gets pain in most parts of her body on most days – a deep ache which gets worse as the day progresses. She experienced aching in her legs and her arms, felt constantly tired, could not remember things very well anymore, never woke up refreshed from sleep and often had episodes of low mood with no real reason.

There is a condition called fibromyalgia syndrome, which, in my opinion, Helen was suffering from. Fibromyalgia syndrome is a poorly understood condition which is thought to be due to widespread dysfunction of the nervous system. We do not know what causes it, but patients complain of diffuse, achy, widespread tenderness throughout all four quadrants of the body. Environmental factors which can trigger fibromyalgia include soft tissue injuries, such as those sustained in a road traffic accident, as well as prolonged periods of psychological stress. The damaged muscles and ligaments from such an accident would normally only result in acute pain lasting for a few weeks, but in a genetically susceptible individual the stress (both from physical injury and psychological distress) can trigger the development of widespread and persistent pain.

Fibromyalgia and other similar conditions such as chronic fatigue syndrome, which fall under the umbrella term of 'central sensitivity syndromes', may be triggered by certain types of infections, for example Lyme disease or viral hepatitis. Psychological stress including deployment to war has also been associated with the development of conditions such as fibromyalgia. There appears to be a mixture of genetic factors that render an individual vulnerable to the development of central sensitivity syndromes. The genetic markers by themselves are not sufficient to cause these conditions but interaction with environmental triggers such as those mentioned above can result in dysfunction of the neurological and hormonal system of the body, producing excitability of the pain system as well as related systems such as those regulating sleep and mood.

Patients with fibromyalgia syndrome have associated sleep disturbance, chronic fatigue and memory impairment. In addition, patients may present with widespread non-specific and confusing (to a myriad of specialties) symptoms that can include bladder dysfunction without any obvious cause, breathlessness without any respiratory disease, dizziness without neurological cause, burning, numbness and tingling unrelated to any nerve injury, irritable bowel syndrome and a host of other symptoms. The diagnosis of fibromyalgia is made using diagnostic criteria where patients score the number of areas that they experience pain in together with the severity of their cognitive impairment, unrefreshing sleep and fatigue. They also score any of the complaints listed above that they suffer with in order to arrive at a composite score. In the absence of any other condition that can better explain their symptoms, and if they meet the threshold score, the patient is given a diagnosis of fibromyalgia syndrome. Fibromyalgia may also occur simultaneously with other chronic pain conditions like osteoarthritis, rheumatoid arthritis and systemic lupus erythematosus. Approximately 10 to 30 per cent of patients with these rheumatic disorders also meet the criteria for a diagnosis of fibromyalgia syndrome.

When I explained this, Helen looked at me fairly sceptically, as most patients do when I talk them through fibromyalgia. In a world where we believe in concrete, visible signs of disease and illness and where there is a scan or blood test for nearly everything, the idea that you can have dysfunctional nerves sounds like psychological gobbledygook to most people. I explained to her that this was quite a lot of information to take in and that she was probably better off reading some of the leaflets that we give to patients about the condition of fibromyalgia syndrome, pain management and the role of clinical psychology in treating it. I offered her the option of coming back to see me if she did not understand the information or, alternatively, if she had understood and wanted to embrace an approach that favoured rehabilitation then she could make an appointment to see one of our clinical psychologists. As first dates go in the pain clinic it was not one of my more successful and I could sense her reticence and her need for a more definitive solution to her problem.

A month passed by and Helen rang the pain service to ask for another appointment. When she sat down, she said to me: 'I do not understand. I do not understand why if my arm is hurting it is not because of a trapped nerve in my neck. I do not understand how I can have pain in my arm that is not due to a trapped nerve or problem with my muscles. Is the pain psychological and are you telling me I am imagining it?' She then started to cry. Her husband leant towards her somewhat helplessly and gently stroked her thigh. When someone starts to cry in clinic I often reflect on the expression 'private pain' and the idea of being alone with your pain. I have never met a lonelier person than someone suffering with pain. Unlike a child that bumps its head and is soothed by the embrace of a parent, the chronic pain sufferer is not helped by the embrace of a loved one because the pain is unrelenting, and you cannot be held all day long.

The body has a system of nerves which form a network and the dysfunction of these nerves results in the experience of persistent pain. I usually google 'nervous system' and use the images section to talk a patient through what they are experiencing. I explain that the nervous system works a bit like a car alarm which goes off because somebody is breaking into the car – this is acute pain and when the car is fixed and the intruders have been chased away the alarm switches off. But sometimes the alarm goes off without there being an intruder and in this case the problem is with the alarm itself. The pain and the loudness of the alarm are both real and not imagined; the problem, however, is not with the machinery but with the way the system functions. Unfortunately, in the case of chronic pain, the alarm cannot be switched off once it is broken – the car owner can only learn to manage their response to the alarm.

This is the most distressing part of my job, offering answers with no hope of a cure. The idea that you have to manage a problem rather than having it cured – there is no disc that can be cut out, no bone that can be mended or joint that can be replaced – is difficult for most people to understand and accept.

I tell Helen that our technology is not yet sufficiently advanced and that there is no scan or blood test which will prove that she has chronic pain. She says her biggest problem is that when she tried to explain fibromyalgia syndrome to her colleagues at work they said, 'Oh, that's a made-up condition, it's all in your head.' Their reaction to her informing them about her chronic pain was to assume she was trying to get out of work. Unfortunately, this kind of negative reaction is not uncommon, even amongst healthcare professionals, and is the result of the widespread lack of understanding around why and how people develop chronic pain.

*

As well as fibromyalgia syndrome, there is also a primary chronic pain syndrome condition called complex regional pain syndrome (CRPS) which deserves special mention.

CRPS is a very unusual condition. It can develop spontaneously or as a result of trauma – for example it could be related to having a fracture or some form of elective surgery – but in either case is characterized by pain that persists after tissue healing has occurred. The first reports of CRPS date back to the reports of Silas Weir Mitchell, a US physician who described the condition in soldiers recovering from gunshot wounds in the American Civil War. The condition has been referred to as Sudeck's atrophy (referring to the thinning of bones seen), reflex sympathetic dystrophy (referring to the changes in colour, temperature and swelling of the affected area) and algodystrophy (from 'algos' meaning pain, 'dys' meaning bad and 'trophy' meaning nourishment, referring to the thinning of bones, blanching of skin and generally sickly looking appearance of the affected limb); the various names reflect the theories which physicians proposed to explain the condition or the predominant symptom observed. The term CRPS was coined in 1995 to resolve the confusion around nomenclature and facilitate further research.

The name given to the condition describes how little we understand about it because it is essentially four words strung together to try to describe something which is still an enigma. The condition is 'complex' and when doctors use this term it implies that they don't understand what something is or why it occurs. It is 'regional' in that it tends to affect an arm or a leg. Pain is a predominant symptom of the condition and usually is present when there shouldn't be a reason for it to persist because the underlying injury is healed, and the pain is 'disproportionate' to the inciting event. Doctors use the word syndrome when they are describing something whose origins they don't understand, but where they are able to identify particular changes and where the patient reports symptoms.

The best way to understand CRPS is to imagine that the usual response of the body to injury – which includes redness, swelling, pain and sensitivity to touch in the injured region – becomes exaggerated and unregulated and persists for longer than is normal. Patients with CRPS develop an abnormal limb which might be hot or cold and changes colour. They may experience a tremor or inhibited movement in the limb that is unrelated to pain and exists because of a dysfunction in the nervous system that we cannot yet explain. They may have loss of hair in the affected region and changes to their skin and nails on that limb; either the nails don't grow as much or overgrow, and the hair is lost from the limb. The symptoms are often florid at the beginning and gradually reduce over time, but the pain persists in 15 per cent of sufferers. Because the condition is so variable it is diagnosed by what are called the Budapest criteria – requiring there to be the changes in colour, swelling, etc. mentioned above in sufficient prominence – so named because the consensus conference to decide on the diagnostic criteria for this condition from a research point of view was held in Budapest in 2010.

The condition is difficult to treat and requires early reha-bilitation. The person needs to have their pain reduced and needs to engage actively with a hand therapist for upper limb CRPS or a physiotherapist if it's the lower limb; spinal cord stimulation, an electrical treatment that we will discuss in Chapter Eight, can also help in terms of reducing the pain. They need to get the limb moving so that they can rewire the nerves and the immune system to dampen down the florid reaction that has occurred due to CRPS in order to facilitate rehabilitation. CRPS is a significant diagnosis when it occurs in the setting of an injury that has a compensation claim attached because the condition renders people considerably disabled, and the literature indicates that in the context of an ongoing medicolegal claim the prognosis for recovery is poor.

CRPS is challenging to diagnose and experts tend to contest a great deal over whether an individual is suffering from it, particularly in medicolegal situations. Sometimes it is florid and even the most ardent defendant-appointed pain expert cannot undermine the diagnosis, but more subtle varieties of CRPS also exist, and often the medical experts are hamstrung by the assessments of the clinicians who have seen the patient and who have not utilized the Budapest criteria when making their assessments.

*

We understand that chronic pain is real pain, it is not imagined, and it is due to nerves which are not working properly. We know that patients with chronic pain do not feel normal and they wake up each day with discomfort. And we also know that disability and pain are not related in the chronic setting. If you break your arm there is a period of time when you cannot use your arm; until it heals you will not have normal function. With chronic pain, however, everything has healed and so what determines your disability is your native resilience in the face of adversity, in the same way that what stops you from managing your diabetes appropriately is not access to healthcare or drugs or the way those drugs work, but your approach to the management of the condition. If you manage it well and maintain your blood sugar within normal levels and choose to eat wisely then you can become prime minister or win four Olympic medals, but if you choose to live badly then the end result will be amputations, dialysis and heart attacks. The difference is not the disease but the way that people approach and manage their condition.

I think it is the fact that people have this choice which sometimes makes it difficult for me in clinic. I love my father. My father is a GP and has been for forty-odd years and still works. I would love my father to live forever. I just had a conversation with him because he went to see his cardiologist, who did the usual stress test and then prescribed yet another drug to lower his cholesterol. However, my dad, who still lives in South Africa, loves fries from the local roadhouse and Bombay mix. He will not change his lifestyle and the only thing that will help him live well and longer is the choices that he makes with regards to Bombay mix and fries. When we love people it is so difficult to deal with the poor choices they make. But when you sit in a pain clinic offering people the opportunity to rehabilitate you are often not privy to their narrative. What role does pain and the disability from pain play in their overall life? How much do they need their Personal Independence Payment as a consequence of their fibromyalgia? What role does their chronic lower-back pain play in maintaining their relationship with their spouse? If they got better would their partners still love them? What is the family dynamic – do they rule the roost with their chronic pain at the centre of attention? Whilst it is the right thing to do from an evidence-based point of view, offering patients rehabilitation as a clinician often completely unseats and unsettles families.

There are three ways to deal with chronic pain. You can spend your time agitating about the alarm going off, you can try to ignore it (but the ignoring of it actually takes up more energy), or the final alternative is to learn to live with this deeply unpleasant situation. There will be times in your life when the alarm is louder, particularly when you are stressed or upset about something else, but there will be times when you busy yourself with other activities and the alarm makes very little difference to your life. Having said this, unlike the management of other chronic conditions such as diabetes or high blood pressure, which you do not feel unless you become acutely unwell, pain is something which is there with you all the time. It demands your attention like a small dog yapping at your heels. It distracts, frustrates and distresses people and affects their identity because if they are constantly being harassed by pain then they cannot accomplish tasks and lay down the memories that make them who they are.

It is not entirely clear to medical science why some people who have an injury or a physical problem go on to develop pain which persists, but we think there are underlying biological reasons. Patients with chronic pain may have different enzymes which predispose them to developing persistent pain; there is an enzyme that breaks down the neurotransmitters noradrenaline and serotonin, chemicals involved in both mood and pain, and people who develop chronic pain have been found to have abnormal versions of these enzymes meaning that they end up with lower levels of these pain-relieving and mood-uplifting chemicals. We also think that psychological factors (thoughts and feelings) can cause physiological changes, particularly changes in brain chemistry, which might lead to a person developing chronic pain, so where a patient is more prone to catastrophizing – magnifying, ruminating and feeling helpless in the face of adversity – this can result in a change in the normal ecosystem of brain connections (the connectome) which then affects the way the muscles and nerves function, and instead of the pain alarm switching off after the body has healed it continues to blare. Genetic factors can also contribute to changes in the way the harm-sensing receptors function. In some individuals they are more abundant and more sensitive, leading to a greater propensity to neural inflammation or prolonged injury. There can also be changes within the connections in the spinal cord, leading to an increase in the number of excitatory chemicals released at the dorsal horn in response to a signal from receptors in the skin and other tissues, causing the spinal cord to become 'wound up' and send more messages to the brain.

The brain itself changes when an individual has developed chronic pain and suffered with it for a long time. The amount of grey matter in the brains of patients with chronic back pain reduces over time and new connections are formed which make the brain more alert and responsive to the experience of pain. It is a bitter irony that the individuals who develop chronic pain become more attuned to feeling pain because of the changes, triggered by pain, which develop in the nervous system that make it even more sensitive. A chronic pain sufferer presenting for surgery that is unrelated to their chronic pain is therefore more likely to experience severe post-operative pain due to this existing dysfunction.

The idea of 'pain stickiness' has been proposed to try to understand why some people develop chronic pain after an injury and others do not – pain sticks because of a host of genetic, environmental, social and psychological factors. We observe physiological changes in individuals suffering chronic pain, such as alterations in nervous system connections in the brain, but we do not yet understand what it means. Ultimately, we yearn for a biobehavioural model to explain why chronic pain develops.

In patients who suffer with catastrophizing thoughts, brain areas are activated which cause the pain pathways to be amplified. When you amplify a pain pathway it is like new channels being formed within a riverbed. Initially there is a trickle of water but as more and more water is released the furrows become wider and wider and eventually they become full raging torrents. This can be, in part, due to behavioural changes that a person makes when they experience pain. Patients who have ruptured their Achilles tendon and are still experiencing pain may think that it has not healed appropriately and may stop walking. If they do this then the tendon may thicken and become immobile. When they then do try to move they experience pain, which reinforces this idea that something is wrong and that the doctors have not fixed it properly. They may see a doctor who does not encourage them to rehabilitate and says to them that the pain should be their guide, whereupon the fact that they continue to experience pain results in them moving even less, aggravating the situation. We now encourage people to rehabilitate in the presence of pain and try to reassure them that theirs is a safe pain; but not every doctor has this paradigm on board, and when such a doctor meets a patient with high levels of pain-related fear then the consequence is increasing disability.

My heart sinks when I come across a patient who says they last worked when Take That first got together because I know that they have a lifestyle which is now ruled by chronic pain. Breaking somebody like this out of the cycle of chronic pain is almost impossible because you are not just trying to manage a clinical problem, you are also threatening to dismantle somebody's world. As a taxpayer and clinician I find myself thinking, 'This patient could be rehabilitated if they only wanted to be,' but then I realize the extent to which our society facilitates chronic pain in so many ways. Persistent pain affects identity formation, which relies on engaging in day-to-day activities. If the society you live in will continue to support you if you adopt a disabled role then it is likely that some people will take this path. As mentioned, chronic pain is not an indicator of tissue damage, and so there are individuals who learn to function despite being accompanied by daily pain, and then there are others who choose to withdraw and are disabled by their pain. This is not always a conscious choice, however.

*

In my ten years as a pain consultant it has become increasingly obvious to me as a doctor that much of what we do in modern medicine is fairly futile – unless we are treating cancers that we can cut out and perhaps prolong life or we are treating trauma or infectious disease. In everything else we are at the wrong point of the thrust of treatment. We should not be the tip of the spear, we should be somewhere on the sides with the tip of the spear being those clinicians who can facilitate and motivate change in the individual and on a wider social scale. When you live in a world that tells you to eat less sugar but then you walk into a supermarket where only two of the aisles actually contain anything nutritious, then you are dealing with a society that is actually up against you in terms of getting people to live well.

The healthcare system, with its doctors, nurses and allied healthcare professionals, hospitals and treatment centres, is constructed on the foundation of being able to arrive at a single diagnosis for a set of complaints and to decree management based on the diagnosis of a disease. Healthcare is an industry (as it has been since the time of Babylon, Ancient Egypt and Greece) and sometimes the maintenance of the industry and status quo becomes more powerful a motivator for the people that work in that industry than alleviating the suffering of the people that the industry was designed to serve. It becomes difficult therefore for the industry to acknowledge its limitations when faced with chronic pain, and rather than attempting a different, non-medicated approach, patients are often passed along from station to station like passengers on a train with no specific destination.

As we have seen in this chapter, chronic pain is incredibly hard to accept for both doctors and patients because the pain is not linked to a 'disease' or injury that can be easily diagnosed with our current technology. There is no blood test or scan that can determine chronic pain. Given these challenges in even diagnosing a chronic pain condition, we will now go on to look at the ways that various medical professions have tried to manage, or even 'cure', chronic pain.

Pain management – needles, narcotics and knives

Whenever I am asked to teach a group of medical students, junior doctors or even a group of my peers, I often quote the words of Marcus Aurelius (the Roman emperor 161–180 AD). He was fond of reminding himself and others that 'everything we hear is an opinion not a fact and everything we see is a perspective not the truth'. Marcus Aurelius was schooled in the philosophy of Stoicism and his *Meditations*, a book recording his private thoughts and a reminder to himself to be humble, patient, empathetic, generous and resolute in the face of adversity, is still widely read today. It is said that he employed somebody to walk beside him whose role was to whisper in his ear, 'You are just a man; you are just a man.'

When it comes to discussing our approach and methods for easing suffering – in medicine generally and in a fledgling field such as pain medicine particularly – I find it helpful to remind myself of Marcus Aurelius's words, that my perspective is but a fleeting moment in time, and that a century from today the procedures that we argue, fuss and fight about will be viewed with a mixture of amusement, curiosity and amazement. Our patterns of thinking, our scientific limitations and hubris, will be reflected on in the same way that we now shake our heads at the physicians who employed bloodletting as a medical panacea, back when illness was believed to be due to an imbalance of the four humours.

The practice of engaging in a trial-and-error approach to therapeutic interventions, with no clear idea of the pathology being treated, is not new in clinical medicine. Our incomplete understanding of disease can lead to ill-conceived interventions which can, today as in centuries past, be responsible for a great deal of harm. Oliver Wendell Holmes, an American Supreme Court Justice in the early twentieth century, is quoted as saying: 'From making the cure of illness more insufferable than the illness itself, Lord deliver us.' It is perhaps also why physicians from antiquity felt the need to state explicitly: *primum non nocere* – first do no harm.

Harm is an interesting concept – it is not always the obvious harm of causing death or paralysis through a misplaced needle, a poorly chosen incision or carelessly used drug. Harm can be facilitating an approach whereby the patient uses your repeat injection procedure to justify their disability and provide a letter to the Department for Work and Pensions. Harm can be that their reliance on your needle causes them not to engage in more effective behaviours such as exercise or mindfulness to manage their pain and disability. Harm can be that you slowly cause their spines to become osteoporotic with repeated steroid injections but so slowly that your injections are not seen as the cause.

Modern interventional techniques to manage pain can, when mishandled, cause harm. They can be broadly broken down into three categories: those that cause destruction of nerves; interventions where therapeutic substances such as local anaesthetics and steroids are injected around joints or nerves; and interventions where electricity is used to stimulate the nervous system (spinal cord stimulation). These techniques fall naturally within the skill set of anaesthesiologists, who are involved in blocking nerves in the perioperative setting to facilitate surgery and in the context of labour wards to relieve the pain of childbirth. Patients with non-specific lower-back pain and patients with peripheral nerve pain (sciatica) due to irritation of spinal nerve roots are therefore easily treated with injection therapies by the same clinicians. There is crossover between the techniques of using a needle and syringe in anaesthesia and that of pain medicine, however in the former the procedure is only done to ensure pain relief for a short while during and after surgery, whereas in pain medicine the condition being treated is fundamentally different.

Modern interventional techniques to manage pain – now slowly being decommissioned in many parts of the world due to a lack of evidence – have relied heavily on the use of steroids. Steroids were first discovered in the 1920s but it was only after the Second World War that patients with rheumatoid arthritis were successfully treated with the steroid cortisone. The spectacular response to steroids in patients with rheumatoid arthritis has made it fundamental to the treatment of inflammatory rheumatological conditions. The powerful inflammatory suppressive nature of steroids led to the application of the substances to what were regarded as inflamed areas of the spine, particularly nerve roots. Initial studies applying steroids to inflamed nerve roots were all carried out on a series of patients, without the randomization of patients with specific diagnoses into treatment and non-treatment groups in order to assess if it was the treatment making the difference or if the result was down to chance. Between 1953 and 1993 most of these studies were retrospective, looking back at patients who had been treated with epidural steroids and then quoting the results. Retrospective studies are famously biased, potentially due to a lack of negative outcomes being recorded. The first prospective studies yielded mixed results. Some showed a striking benefit from epidural steroid injection whilst others showed the injection of steroids to be no more effective than a placebo injection in relieving chronic symptoms caused by proven lumbar disc herniation. Despite this very weak evidence base the practice of epidural steroid injection into the spine continues today.

There was a time before the Nuremberg Code (1947) and the Declaration of Helsinki (1964) and the advent of evidence-based medicine, when doctors experimented freely without having to conduct ethically approved, carefully constructed studies, overseen by committees and aimed at identifying the treatment effect of an intervention (the actual effect minus the placebo effect) and evaluating its safety. Lumbar facet joints, which are the sliding joints between the bones of the spine, were first described as a possible source of back pain in 1911, and the term facet joint syndrome was coined in 1933. In order to understand if back pain was originating in these joints a so-called 'provocative' study was undertaken (as opposed to a 'therapeutic' study) by a team of doctors led by C. Hirsch in 1963. His team injected saltwater, which is a highly irritant substance, into the facet joints of volunteers, inducing pain in the lower back, sacroiliac and gluteal areas, and studied the results in their paper entitled 'Studies on pain following injections of hypertonic saline in discs, joints and ligaments in the low back':

In order to check the different cartilaginous and ligamentous elements as to the symptoms they may cause, when subjected to irritation, hypertonic solution of saline 0.1% was injected in the following way. One thin long needle was introduced between the spinous processes transdurally into the fourth or fifth, or both lumbar discs in patients with low back pain. Another needle was placed on one of the lower intervertebral joints. Positions were checked by X-ray in AP and lateral views. The patients were in a prone position and were not under any anaesthesia. Less than 0.3 ml was injected into the vertebral joint. Pain occurred after a few seconds and was very annoying.

The first recorded therapeutic injection of the facet joints with steroid and local anaesthetics was done by two ortho-paedic surgeons, Vert Mooney and James Robertson, in 1976, followed by a radiologist I. W. McCall and his team in 1979, bringing this therapy into increasingly widespread use for lower-back pain over the next thirty years until its recent evaluation as not being of any benefit.

There is controversy surrounding who the first person was to inject substances into the epidural space to treat patients with pain; credit is given to the French neurolo-gist Jean-Athanase Sicard (1872–1929), however around the same time a physician called Fernand Cathelin (1873–1960), also from Paris, had been treating patients with epidural injections for several months. The first series of nine patients who underwent epidural injections included a patient suffering with syphilis that had invaded the nervous system, four patients suffering with lower-back pain and four patients with pain due to nerve injury. Sicard, who per-formed these procedures, became famous as a pain doctor during the First World War when he used alcohol to destroy peripheral nerves in order to alleviate pain, particularly in conditions such as complex regional pain syndrome. Perhaps it was because he published his ideas in the French language that they were not widely read, however, and the idea of using the epidural route to help with pain did not spread as quickly as other medical innovations. We would refer to this phenomenon today as publication bias and it continues to thwart medical progress. What is curious about the technique is that the disease which we most commonly use epidural steroid injections for today (as opposed to epidurals used for pain relief after surgery and during childbirth), which is herniated discs causing compression or irritation of nerves commonly referred to as sciatica, was not widely known until 1934 – it is quite possible therefore that patients who responded to the therapy happened to be suffering with sciatica and their serendipitous response promoted the therapy.

Controversy exists around whether the American neurologist James Corning or the German surgeon August Bier was the first to perform a spinal anaesthetic. Spinal anaesthetics, or subarachnoid blocks, differ from epidural injections in that the epidural space is separated from the subarachnoid space by the dura (hence the 'epi-dural' space). The cerebrospinal fluid flows in the subarachnoid space and anything injected here has direct access to the nerves of the spinal cord rather than just the nerves *exiting* the spinal cord, as in the case of an epidural injection. In 1885 Corning injected cocaine into the intrathecal (around the spinal cord) space of a man who was diagnosed as suffering with habituated masturbation and seminal incontinence; the long-term outcome of the treatment is not known. In 1898 August Bier performed a spinal anaesthetic, injecting

15 mg of cocaine into the fluid surrounding the spinal cord, and successfully anaesthetized one of his resident patients, August Hildebrandt, having previously used the technique on a series of six patients. He tested the effect of the local anaesthetic on Hildebrandt by checking loss of sensation in response to the application of a burning cigar to the skin, a strong blow to the shin with an iron hammer and strong pressure and traction on one of the testicles. We tend not to use these methods today, preferring the application of ethyl chloride which is felt as a cold sensation when it evaporates from the skin; patients who have had a local anaesthetic introduced into the cerebral spinal fluid feel the sensation as warm or not at all.

Local anaesthetic introduced to the intrathecal or sub-arachnoid space is used for operations performed below the belly button, including Caesarean sections, but this space is limited in terms of its usefulness regarding chronic pain. Intrathecal drug delivery using very low dose local anaes-thetic, opioids or conotoxin (a neurotoxin derived from the sea snail *Conus magus*) to block the calcium channels in nerves can be used to treat chronic pain, using an implanted pump that is periodically refilled. The helpfulness of this therapy, however, is limited, and complications associated with the technique have made it unpopular. In cancer pain, substances such as alcohol or phenol are sometimes used to destroy nerves using the intrathecal route but only when life expectancy is less than the time that it would take for nerves to start regenerating, which would cause more severe pain.

The evolution of interventional pain therapies blossomed from the therapeutic tradition of offering patients with intractable cancer pain relief from their suffering through destructive neurosurgical and anaesthetic procedures, prior to the gradual development of more effective oncology therapies and holistic palliative care services in the latter part of the twentieth century. There was an acceptance of these destructive therapies because patients often did not live very long, and the long-term complications from destroying nerves were often not experienced – the patient would succumb before manifesting the pain from regenerating nerves or the ignominy of incontinence. Some nerve-destruction techniques are still practised today such as cordotomies, first performed in 1912, where the pain pathways at the level of the cervical spinal cord are destroyed in patients who have pain on one side of their body. This is an invasive therapy with potentially severe complications, but it does offer individuals with relatively short life expectancies relief from pain and suffering. Similarly the nerve supply to the pancreas can be destroyed by injecting alcohol, phenol or glycerol into the bundle of nerves accessing this organ, disrupting the normal architecture of the nerves by dissolving protective fat layers and obliterating the orderly sodium and potassium channels on the surface of the nerve which enable electricity to flow. But unlike distinct fibre optic cables transmitting discrete packets of information, nerves are intermingled and inseparable, and the destruction of nerves which transmit pain also unfortunately disrupts nerves that control the function of the gut, causing diarrhoea, bladder and bowel incontinence and paralysis of the legs.

These therapies are now used more infrequently and judiciously because cancer survival rates are greater, and we rely much more on painkillers and anti-cancer drugs to manage cancer pain. Because nerves regenerate when you destroy them with glycerol and alcohol, and the regenerating nerve expresses new sodium and potassium channels in a haphazard fashion when they do regenerate, the long-term consequences of nerve destruction are then worse than the pain they were originally designed to treat. The new channels act like the frayed end of a ruptured electrical cable, sparking, burning and fizzing as they desperately try to conduct electrically encoded information to the section of nerve that they have been separated from. This is called deafferentation pain. Techniques using alcohol, phenol or glycerol to destroy nerves are therefore not appropriate for patients who suffer with chronic non-malignant or chronic non-cancer related pain. These patients are likely to live for a long time and using techniques such as glycerol would result in worse neuropathic pain in the years following the procedure.

Interventional techniques using needles to reach nerve bundles evolved over time to be incorporated into the specialty of anaesthesiology. As medical specialties became more evolved, with palliative medicine taking over the care of cancer sufferers from a symptom-management point of view, anaesthesiologists working in pain medicine migrated more towards treating non-malignant pain with similar techniques using steroids and local anaesthetics but which did not result in destruction of nerves, thus circumventing the issue of deafferentation pain. It is interesting to note that the techniques and the application of novel therapeutic substances preceded any theory of why the person had pain, rather than the other way around. Albert Einstein was particularly critical of any approach where technique evolves before theoretical explanation and Sir Arthur Conan Doyle, himself a physician, expressed through his fictional character Sherlock Holmes his suspicion of the approach of theorizing before one possesses data, as this would, in his view, lead to twisting facts to suit theories rather than using facts to develop theories.

The focus for anaesthesiologists involved in treating chronic pain throughout the twentieth century was on pain relief rather than curing the underlying condition which (most) clinicians soon realized was not possible. Many pain clinics largely ignored or were ill-equipped or -motivated to incorporate behavioural and physiotherapy treatments to manage the loss of function which patients with persistent pain suffered with, as well as the psychological distress which followed from this loss of the ability to work and perform the activities of daily living. Millions of pounds have therefore been spent on the injection of local anaesthetic and steroids into lumbar facet joints as well as epidural steroid injections over the last fifty years, despite questionable value to patients and a very poor platform for their usefulness from a theoretical or evidence-based point of view. This century has seen a shift to more managed healthcare with greater involvement of the organizations, both public and private, that pay for treatments with a rigorous assessment of the cost versus benefit of treatments and the scientific evidence which underpins the therapy.

Whilst the interventional pain medicine doctors from an anaesthetic background have been happily flying solo, injecting patients with local anaesthetic and steroid, burning nerves and prescribing drugs, there has been a parallel evolution in the understanding of chronic pain as a disease rather than merely a symptom, where the chronification of pain is understood to be due to a complex dysfunction of the nervous system. There has been and continues to be a surreal disregard by some doctors of the complexity of chronic pain and the influence of psychological and social factors on its maintenance and evolution and the myriad pathways to and from the spinal cord that influence the experience of pain – be it acute pain due to injury, or chronic pain, either cancerous or non-cancerous. Anaesthesiologists who practise in the field of pain medicine and perform interventions are often labelled 'needle jockeys' by psychologists and pain management physiotherapists, who marvel at the obliviousness of the individual wielding the needle to the psychological distress of the patient, and at the limited literature on the safety, efficacy, fiscal neutrality and effectiveness of interventional pain techniques.

There is a great deal of expressed and hidden anger on the part of psychologists and pain management physiotherapists, as well as occupational therapists and nurses who work in pain medicine, with regards to the amount of money that has been poured into interventional techniques. This does lead to very interesting (and infrequent) meetings of multidisciplinary pain societies, and I sometimes wonder if this ability by most pain anaesthesiologists to ignore the widely available literature on the complexity of chronic pain is deliberate or whether it merely stems from the absolute belief in their own abilities in terms of relieving pain. Are they continuing to provide these therapies because they only ever see their benefit at the six-week mark when the patient is reviewed in their clinic? Are they perfectly happy to accept that the provision of a therapy which only has a short-term benefit is justifiable even in the absence of collecting data with regards to possible long-term side effects? The ongoing provision of injection therapies to patients with chronic non-cancer pain and the patient's silent (to the doctor) descent into a vortex of disability is perhaps best illustrated with Diane's story.

*

Diane had a difficult and troubled childhood, responding with displays of anger and anxiety to the conflict between her parents. Her father divorced her mother when she was sixteen and the family were forced to move far away from Diane's circle of friends and social support structures. When she was in her twenties, she suffered with frequent headaches and a strain to her lower back. She also presented to her GP with abdominal pain that could never be pinned down to a specific disease and complained bitterly about painful periods.

Her lower back started to hurt during her first pregnancy and, as the months during her pregnancy progressed, her backache became worse. Her pain resolved after the birth of her child but returned when she had her second child. In her early thirties the back pain became continuous. She found her job as a cleaner unrewarding and the management were unsympathetic towards her with regards to her pain and the limitations it placed on her ability to work. She sought help from her GP, who prescribed codeine and paracetamol to help her symptoms. He was unable to provide her with an explanation of why she had lower-back pain, dismissing it as a common occurrence in people who did manual work, but he performed an examination to rule out anything dangerous in the form of a tumour or a fracture of her spine. She had full control of her bladder and bowel function, so he was not worried that she had a disc prolapse compressing the nerves radiating from her spinal cord. The persistence of her back pain and her associated distress led to a referral by the GP to an orthopaedic service where she was seen by a nurse. The nurse explained that the pain Diane was experiencing was coming from her sacroiliac joint, which is an immovable joint between the hips and the sacrum (a triangular bone in the lower back).

Diane continued to complain of back pain and increasingly found that it was interfering with her ability to work and disrupting her sleep. She felt generally unwell – tired, achy, lethargic and depressed. By the time she was in her late thirties her pain had become so continuous and limiting that she stopped working. Her GP continued to treat her symptoms with increasingly strong medication and eventually she was started on morphine.

Diane was eventually referred to a pain clinic where she met an anaesthesiologist with a subspecialty interest in pain medicine, who worked in a clinic without a psychologist or physiotherapist. In his view, after prodding her cursorily for five minutes, she had pain emanating from the sacroiliac joint and he listed her for injection of this joint. He injected local anaesthetic and steroid as a day procedure, using an X-ray machine to guide the needle into the joint, which sounds wonderfully technical and not surprisingly has a tremendous placebo effect.

Unfortunately but not unpredictably, the injection into Diane's lower back and into the sacroiliac joint only gave her five weeks' pain relief, but the pain consultant considered this to be a positive outcome and listed her for radiofrequency denervation of the nerve supplying the joint, which means he planned to insert a needle into the nerve and apply a radiofrequency wave which would excite the ions within the nerve, destroying it on a semi-permanent basis. Diane continued to seek answers from her GP when her pain continued despite these interventions, but he still could not furnish her with an understanding of why she had persistent pain. When the sacroiliac joint injection did not improve her symptoms her pain consultant moved on to other joints within the lumbar region of her spine, performing first local anaesthetic and steroid injections into the facet joints followed up by procedures to burn the nerve giving sensation to these joints. He then performed an epidural injection – bathing the nerves that leave the spine in a mixture of local anaesthetic and steroid.

Diane's injection journey continued for a year, at the end of which she was on a disability living allowance and no longer able to do her own housework. When the pain consultant had run out of sites to inject, he referred Diane to physiotherapy for an assessment and finally discharged her to a community pain management service which was run by a psychologist and a physiotherapist.

Diane's story follows a common theme. Episodes of acute non-specific lower-back pain beginning in pregnancy and transforming into persistent pain is not an unusual story. We think that these episodes of acute pain hammer away at the pain alarm system, eventually rendering it permanently active by changing connections in the brain and spinal cord. Diane had several psychological factors in the form of anxiety and depression making her vulnerable to the development of chronic pain as well as environmental factors which have impacted on her nervous system slowly, damaging it with an unfavourable chemical environment – like cigarette smoking which over the years nagged at cells in the lungs causing bouts of inflammation and infection and would eventually lead to cancerous transformation or persistent breathlessness. The service she was referred to applied treatments in line with those practised by pain clinics across the world, present in both public and private health services. Diane said that these consultations never lasted long and always ended with her either receiving the promise of a cure from an injection or being referred back to her GP for further medication management.

*

The outcome measure to judge the success of an intervention may be considered simply to be a reduction in pain, rather than whether pain reduction results in improved function and psychological well-being. The pain centre I work at is very active and mindful in appreciating the growing body of evidence with regards to the biological, psychological and social factors influencing persistent pain conditions. I sometimes feel, however, when I go to meetings and sit in the company of clinicians committed to cure at the end of a needle, that I am sitting alone on the outside of an interventional pain medicine town when it comes to the way that I practise pain medicine.

In October 2018 I attended a meeting of interventional pain doctors considered experts in their field. The group of clinicians were hosted in a chateau in Fontenay-Trésigny in the heart of the Brie region in France, and the meeting was organized and hosted by a company that manufactures the equipment used for interventional pain techniques, including the machine used to ablate nerves – one of the techniques tried, unsuccessfully, on Diane. Injection of local anaesthetic and steroid around facet joints only gives the patient approximately three to six months' pain relief at best, and so the idea evolved that if you use radio waves to burn the nerve which supplies sensation to these joints then the pain relief will be more permanent – this is nerve ablation. This nerve runs over the transverse process of a vertebral body. If you imagine a narrow stream running over a craggy rock in the middle of a mountain, and now imagine you have to access this target with a fine needle inserted from beyond the stratosphere, then it might give you some idea of the complexity of the technique. It is very easy to miss the water but quite easy to hit a structure adjacent to the water which may result in significant complications.

The assembled group of experts were discussing how to insert the needle and whether using X-ray or ultrasound to guide the needle was more appropriate. The amount of heat generated by the needle tip as well as whether this was a pulsed or continuous radiofrequency was discussed at length. I suggested to the assembled group that we did not even understand the nature of the disease we were trying to treat, nor did we have an understanding of its pathological or anatomical basis, and therefore discussions about the techniques of specific therapies appeared to be premature and ludicrous given what we already know about the short-term benefit of these therapies, the lack of long-term benefit and the potential for complications such as nerve damage.

They agreed grudgingly with the logic of my statement. There was a reluctant admission that we have got ourselves into a real fix as pain experts. We have failed over the years to collect the evidence concerning which patients do benefit from this therapy. There is no doubt that some patients do derive pain relief from interventional pain therapies such as radiofrequency ablation of the nerve that supplies sensation to the facet joints. There are also patients who benefit from local anaesthetic and steroid injections, if only on a temporary basis but enough to facilitate rehabilitation – enabling them to walk a little further, change their bedding and wash the dishes. We don't understand the precise mechanism of why these therapies should work in a chronic pain condition where pain persists due to changes in the way the nerves function. Is it the placebo effect, whereby the patient believes they will experience pain relief, and chemicals are therefore released in the brain that block pain signals? Does our meddling perhaps activate the patient's native descending inhibitory pain pathways? Or is it something that happens on a cellular level?

We have failed as a specialty to identify the exact nature of the kind of pain which is responsive to these injections. As a result, the evidence broadly points to them being of very low utility in the management of non-specific lower-back pain. Those responsible for paying for healthcare (governments and private health insurers) are therefore now refusing to fund these treatments, and the result is that the groups of patients who *do* benefit from these procedures, usually the elderly, are now being excluded along with those patients for whom the application of the therapy was inappropriate.

*

In chronic pain, curing the abnormal nervous system is not feasible given our current understanding of pain (or lack of) and therefore our ability to design effective treatments is thwarted by our infantile grasp of the complexities of the alarm system. What is more feasible and important at this stage is attempting to help the sufferer alter their behavioural response to the pain alarm. To take a common example, when it comes to lower-back pain, we do not have the drugs or the interventional pain therapies that can permanently modulate the pain. We have made some progress with modulating pain from damaged nerves in the form of spinal cord stimulators, but the management of non-specific lower-back pain remains elusive. In the meantime, this condition places an enormous burden on society leading to massive losses in economic activity. Whilst we cannot 'cure' it, what we can do is help people understand that these abnormal sensations are not dangerous and teach them to successfully live with persistent pain. Unfortunately, we have not designed the healthcare services with this ethos in mind.

What we have done is to create pain clinics consisting largely of doctors drawn from an anaesthetic background who attempt to make a diagnosis based on a philosophy that aims to attribute a complex condition to a problem within a single structure, such as a facet joint; this philosophy is rooted in the old Cartesian model of pain, which you may remember from Chapter two. This approach leads to inferring a relationship between changes on a patient's MRI scan and the pain that they experience, despite the fact that the changes visible will in fact occur in as many people untroubled by pain as they do in people with persistent pain. If you scan a thirty-year-old who has no back pain, the MRI will show all the same changes associated with somebody who has back pain. There is therefore little basis for making a connection from a pathological point of view between a scan and an individual's pain, because the changes occur just as frequently in people without pain.

Unfortunately, as a specialty we have continued to perform these interventionalist procedures and amass the fees for them, creating an industry with treatments that we can market and sell. At the meeting in Fontenay-Trésigny I was told by one of the company representatives that nobody could understand why doctors from a certain country could perform so many procedures during a session. They then found out that these doctors would bring the patient back on three occasions rather than doing the full procedure at one sitting. The reason for this apparent productivity was purely about collecting triple the fee.

The National Institute for Health and Care Excellence (NICE) in the UK has now issued guidance with regards to the management of lower-back pain, curtailing the use of interventional pain therapies based on the available evidence. NICE is the government body that evaluates therapies used in the National Health Service in terms of whether the therapy offered has an evidence base and guides clinicians with regards to service implementation. These agreements regarding interventional pain therapies were reached with great difficulty due to the vast vested interests at play with regards to the management of non-specific lower-back pain. Whilst in the UK NICE has taken charge, through commissioning groups, of what services can be provided, in the rest of the world it is still very much like the Wild West, where somebody can go on a course over a weekend and then be burning nerves in someone's back on the Monday. Because doctors make a living from performing procedures, these continue to be offered despite little evidence upon which to base them and an incomplete understanding of the condition for which they are used. This goes against the age-old advice of the Greeks with which we started this chapter: *primum non nocere* – first do no harm.

Many pain physicians reading this will probably be quite irritated and annoyed. I have done all these procedures which I have discussed, and I have followed patients up at length and I do appreciate that in some individuals these methods may well reduce chronic non-malignant pain. I know, however, that in the long term these interventions do not improve function, nor do they reduce the distress associated with not understanding why pain has persisted. In my view, when dealing with younger patients repeated interventional techniques leads to collusion between the pain physician and the sufferer of chronic pain by validating the condition and facilitating disability. Patients like Diane are left no better off following multiple interventions which can span a year or more. Diane was left more disabled, more distressed, with less understanding of her chronic pain and caught in a spiral of worsening distress and disability. All I have tried to do in this chapter is to highlight the fact that, in the face of such distress, it is quite easy as a doctor to offer a therapy in the absence of robust outcome measures.

Doctors in all parts of the world are at the tip of the spear when it comes to the management of chronic non-cancer pain. In my opinion this is a fundamental flaw in the system, because reducing the distress and disability associated with chronic pain – which is essentially a condition that cannot be cured – does not rely on the skills of doctors. This is not a condition where there is a broken bone that needs to be plated and fixed and where knowledge about the anatomy of the arm and the correct use of a plate and screws is essential. It is also not a condition where we have appropriate and accurate tests to diagnose the degree of pathology and prescribe medications to manage the disturbance. Chronic pain management is not diabetes, which consists of assessing the degree of blood sugar control that an individual has and carefully titrating insulin to produce a blood sugar within normal range. This type of disease management is what doctors are good at, and that is why we learn physiology, pharmacology and anatomy at medical school. Even in a condition as clear-cut as diabetes, once the doctor has done their initial job the role of psychologists and nurses is in fact more important because maintaining compliance with regards to the condition is much more impactful long term than any changes in medication.

Pain medicine is a fascinating example of a specialty that has never really come to grips with the nature of the condition it seeks to cure, but which has ploughed ahead with the application of therapies borrowed from other specialties in order to justify its existence. Anaesthesiologists involved in pain medicine have piggybacked on various revolutions, including the fashion of treating acute pain aggressively with opioid therapy and using steroids applied to the spine to treat chronic non-cancer pain.

Interventional pain medicine is a perfect example of how an industry can be built around poor science and dubious data. As a branch of medicine it has evolved from incomplete models and entrenched beliefs related to a complex phenomenon. The rush to action in the face of suffering has come before careful consideration of the evidence; therapies have been accepted without critical evaluation and because they do not appear to cause obvious harm their practice has continued. A more complete approach is needed that represents an intersecting Venn diagram of needles, knives, analgesics and interdisciplinary rehabilitation aimed at behavioural change, with the intersection of the diagram being a reduction in the distress and disability associated with persistent pain.

A journey of a
thousand miles...

Patients who present with intractable chronic pain do not 'fit' into a neat diagnostic label and are like people who arrive by train at a frontier town in the old Wild West. The pain clinic is often their 'last chance saloon' stop on a journey which has passed through many cities and many different specialties – several of which we explored in the previous chapter. Patients have often been subjected to numerous treatments and investigations on the way to the pain clinic and arrive confused, wary, weary and desperate, like survivors of an apocalypse or entrepreneurs who have lost fortunes and optimism at the different stations on their journey to cure and understand their chronic pain. Patients with back pain may, for example, have been reviewed by neurosurgeons or spinal orthopaedic surgeons, with no explanation being provided for their ongoing symptoms. The time spent at these stations has often resulted in increased distress, as they are promised therapies which ultimately do not relieve their symptoms or, even worse, make them feel that they are amongst the incurable and must live with the knowledge that their condition will continue to progress, that they are cursed with ever-increasing disability. Many come to believe that a life spent in a wheelchair is their only future.

On their journey they may have encountered pain physicians who believe that the sufferer of chronic pain can be helped with a single intervention. These are the mavericks of the frontier town promising a magic bullet – one injection or tablet that will resolve the unpleasantness which the person is experiencing and restore them to fully functioning members of society. Then there are other pain physicians living in the frontier town who live on the other side of the tracks, of whom I am one, who believe that the problems that the chronic pain patient suffers with are more complex and require greater input from a wider variety of people. These are the reformed gunslingers who now work collaboratively with psychologists and physiotherapists in order to reduce the distress and disability associated with persistent pain, understanding that the gunslinger misses more often than he hits, that sometimes the bullet may cause unintended harm and that violence is not the answer. Hope and desperation are the baggage accompanying patients with persistent pain as they disembark from the train, and this makes them vulnerable to promises of a therapy involving a single intervention that will facilitate a cure.

One of the phrases that patients with persistent pain

often use in clinic and which makes my heart sink whenever I hear it is, 'I will try anything, Doctor.' This statement usually implies a desperate passivity ('Do something to me, Doctor. Fix me.') and a lack of active engagement by the patient in their management and care. Patients get to a point where they will cling on to any fragment of poorly constructed hope or wild explanation of the cause of their pain, due to desperation and a belief in the power of the doctor to mend their broken bodies. We often collude with patients as doctors by not emphasizing the changes in behaviour which need to take place to improve health. The equivalent example is presenting yourself to a gym but not acknowledging that you will have to change your diet or turn up regularly to achieve the benefits.

For many patients a pain clinic is their final and often reluctant destination. The route to reach the pain clinic has often been meandering, with patients moving between orthopaedic and spinal surgeons, with detours to neurosurgeons and often to pain clinics that have only offered interventions, as opposed to any rehabilitation. This journey only adds to the distress with which individuals present. Some arrive with a weary resignation and a hopeless despair and are perhaps more easily inspired to change and be educated about chronic pain, whilst others arrive angry and spoiling for a fight because of the failure of the doctors they have seen to restore them to normal health. The latter are often caught in a vortex of disability from which they do not feel that they can escape.

Pain and suffering are intimately related. Patients who experience persistent unpleasant body sensations are often faced with fear, anxiety and depression. Pain behaviour is another component of the concept of pain and refers to those things that people say and do when they are suffering. These behaviours are a way for the individual to communicate their pain, distress and suffering. If you want to understand somebody's perception of pain and their response to these abnormal sensations then it is essential that their experience as a whole is considered: an examination of the biological changes potentially underpinning the pain such as inflammation, along with any psychological factors and the society and cultural environment within which the individual finds themselves. If you only focus on one of these aspects – biological, psychological or social – then the formulation of the problem that the person is suffering with will be inadequate and any attempts to manage chronic pain and associated distress and disability will inevitably result in failure.

The preceding chapter discussed the inadequacies of trying to manage chronic pain purely as if the problem was biological, without any acknowledgement of the psychosocial factors involved – finding a target and obliterating it with a needle-based intervention. This chapter outlines an approach which integrates all facets of pain. The aim of pain management programmes is to enable people with chronic pain to achieve as normal a life as possible by reducing physical disability and emotional distress.

*

Patients who come to my pain clinic can be grouped into three broad categories based on the biological mechanism of their pain. First, there are patients who suffer with pain due to disease or injury of a nerve (neuropathic pain). Of these, the most common group is patients who have had a prolapse of an intervertebral disc with consequent compression of nerves as they leave the spinal canal. This causes the condition colloquially called sciatica and is experienced as a sharp shooting pain radiating down the leg (when the compressed nerve is in the lower spine) or arm (when the compression of the nerve is in the neck) which is innervated by the damaged nerve. Patients have often had surgery to decompress the nerve, however the pain persists due to the irreversible damage done to the nerve by the compression combined with an as-yet-unknown genetic predisposition to the development of chronic pain. Patients therefore complain of both leg and back pain since some of the branches of this nerve also provide sensation to the lower back, and abnormal postures adopted due to leg pain can give rise to musculoskeletal back pain.

Other causes of neuropathic pain include trigeminal neuralgia, which affects the nerves of the face and jaw, and patients who have had nerve damage due to diabetes or multiple sclerosis (autoimmune damage to the brain and spinal cord), but these groups of patients are much smaller in number. Neuropathic pain is difficult to treat using the coping strategies that are delivered in the context of a pain management programme because of the episodic, unpredictable and disruptive nature of the pain.

The second group of patients who attend the pain clinic consists of those who suffer with nociplastic pain due to episodes of inflammation from trauma or rheumatological diseases. These diseases involve dysfunction of the immune system where the body tries to digest itself. Repeated episodes of inflammation result in an increasing sensitivity of the pain alarm. Patients experience a constant level of background pain punctuated by flare-ups of pain when their disease is out of control. We occasionally see patients in this category with conditions such as rheumatoid arthritis or psoriatic arthropathy, but they are a very small part of our practice.

The third, and by far the largest, group of patients who are suitable for and potentially benefit from pain management rehabilitation are those who suffer with non-specific chronic lower-back pain and patients who suffer with chronic widespread pain, usually in the form of conditions such as fibromyalgia syndrome, as we saw in Helen's case in Chapter Five. These patients tend to participate in either individual sessions of pain management rehabilitation with a physiotherapist and a psychologist or go on to take part in a pain management programme based on group cognitive behavioural therapy.

*

The pain management centre in which I work has evolved a process for assessing patients which begins prior to them being seen in clinic and attempts to outline the individual's problem within the context of a biopsychosocial model. We receive referrals from many sources; letters that have been written by the stationmasters at the various train stations that the individuals have already visited. Most commonly, patients are referred by their GP or by the GP at the request of a hospital doctor such as an orthopaedic spinal surgeon or neurosurgeon. We assess these referrals and usually prioritize patients who have cancer pain or where the person is at risk of losing their job. Where referrals indicate that the person has not been fully investigated and that there are outstanding medical issues which have not been resolved, particularly when they have ongoing appointments with other clinicians, then we write back to the referrer to explain that it is unlikely that an individual will accept the model we are proposing if they do not feel they have visited all possible stations to explore those options. When a decision has been made to accept the referral, we send out a pack of questionnaires for the patient to complete at home.

The questionnaires that we use include a narrative component where the person is asked about the onset of their pain, which often becomes very relevant if their pain started after an accident for which there is an ongoing medicolegal claim. The medicolegal process is stressful and involves multiple appointments which will have an impact on the person's ability to engage with the service because the ongoing claim can impact significantly on their response to rehabilitation. Patients often experience a great deal of anger if their persistent pain is due to an accident or event which was beyond their control – and that anger exacerbates and maintains pain.

We ask patients about:

- the sites and nature of their pain as well as the duration of their symptoms;
- the clinicians whom they have seen before and the treatments that they have had under these clinicians in the past;
- medication that they are currently receiving or have received, and their opinion of the medication in terms of whether they find painkillers of benefit or have experienced negative drug effects;
- whether they are is in the process of being interviewed for the purposes of being assigned disability payments, if there is a medicolegal claim or if they are undergoing stressful tribunal processes associated with benefits;
- whether they smoke or drink, as this has an impact on pain and is indicative of potentially unhelpful behaviours related to the management of illness;
- what their expectations of the pain centre are and what their current understanding of their pain is.

This latter section is often the most revealing and the responses vary from 'I have no expectations' to pages and pages of ideas, concerns and expectations related to the experience of pain. We also include a diagram of the human body and ask the patient to indicate where their pain is and what sensations they are feeling. Responses here vary from a single X placed over the entire body to finely detailed and multicoloured annotations indicating various pains. The diagram is useful particularly when we are looking at patients with neuropathic pain, where a detailed diagram indicating numbness, tingling or burning in the distribution of the affected nerve is often a helpful indicator of a specific nerve injury.

The questionnaire attempts to capture the patient's level of distress and disability as well as the thought patterns they have with regards to their experience of pain. The free-text element of the questionnaire covers the biological, psychological and social aspects of the impact of their experience of pain. The psychometric tests we administer in the questionnaire attempt to do the same but in a more standardized and scientific manner in order to compare patients and stratify them according to levels of distress and disability. These tests measure pain severity and interference, depression, anxiety, difficulty with performing activities, catastrophizing, fear of movement and quality of life.

The questionnaire tries to outline the patient's degree of disability related to pain. They are given a series of questions to answer including whether they change position frequently to try to get comfortable, what impact pain has on their ability to walk and dress as well as turn over in bed. Patients complete a Brief Pain Inventory, which consists of a series of questions that ask them, on a scale of zero to ten, where zero is no pain and ten is the worst pain they can imagine, what their worst pain has been in the past twenty-four hours and likewise the least amount of pain. We also ask patients where their pain ranks on average and how much relief medications or other treatments have provided in the past twenty-four hours. The Brief Pain Inventory also has a pain interference scale, where zero indicates no interference with daily life, and ten equals complete interference; patients are asked to rate on this scale how much pain interferes with their general activity, mood, walking ability, normal work (including both work outside the home and housework), their relations with other people, sleep and enjoyment of life. We can compare the patient's score with a group of individuals who have presented to the pain clinic before and the levels of rehabilitation intervention required can be inferred to some degree from this comparison.

As part of the questionnaire patients rate their perceived quality of life on a scale from very poor to very good. Pain impacts on function and loss of function results in low mood; one section of the questionnaire therefore seeks to quantify the degree of depression which the individual experiences, including questions such as: 'Over the last two weeks have you had little interest or pleasure in doing things or felt down, depressed and hopeless?' 'Have you had trouble falling or staying asleep or feel tired and have had little energy?' This section also tends to include enquiries about appetite and concentration. One of the questions specifically asks about the risk of suicide, and where patients admit to feeling that they would want to harm themselves nearly every day it triggers a letter to their GP to inform them of this potential risk. Patients who suffer with persistent pain may have minimal to severe depression, and co-morbid pre-existing depression and anxiety can play a significant role. The presence of moderately severe to severe depression significantly compromises the individual's ability to take on board information and initiate the change needed to successfully manage their pain.

The presence of persistent pain understandably makes people very anxious. Patients are afraid of the reasons behind their continued experience of pain and can develop pain-related fear. When assessing pain-related fear we administer a psychometric questionnaire that specifically explores different kinds of fears and anxieties related to pain. Patients may experience physiological disturbances due to the experience of pain: their heart may begin to pound or race, or they may begin trembling when engaged in an activity that increases pain. Where patients experience this internal derangement and disquiet due to the experience of pain it results in the release of neurotransmitters that further sensitize the pain alarm system.

Some patients experience cognitive anxiety due to the experience of pain and are constantly thinking about pain, making them unable to concentrate. Others stop using the body part they perceive their pain to be coming from, which leads to behavioural deconditioning and physical deactivation, and can spiral the individual into disability. Avoiding movement is a natural reaction to pain – but whilst this is reasonable when the pain will resolve within a few weeks it is unhelpful when pain persists. Muscles and joints stiffen due to inactivity and movement then causes further pain which reinforces fear of movement.

The most common understanding of pain is that it is due to undiagnosed injury. Patients believe that pain is a guide and that the experience of pain when moving is a sign that they are making the situation worse. We appreciate that this is not the case in chronic pain, as previously explained, but the presence of high levels of fear of movement (kinesiophobia), severely impacts on a person's ability to function. We therefore administer a specific questionnaire to establish the degree of kinesiophobia which the individual experiences. The patient is given a number of statements to which they respond by either strongly disagreeing, somewhat disagreeing, somewhat agreeing or strongly agreeing, for example: 'I'm afraid that I might injure myself if I exercise', 'My body is telling me that I have something dangerously wrong', 'Pain always means I have injured my body', 'Being careful that I do not make any unnecessary movements is the safest thing I can do to prevent my pain from worsening'. The ultimate score indicates the degree of kinesiophobia.

Finally, we also administer a score which tries to quantify the patient's level of catastrophizing. Patients who catastrophize to a high degree require intensive psychological input to alter their belief systems and natural ways of coping.

The completed questionnaire, made up of the patient's free-text answer and their responses to the various psychometric tests outlined above, gives us an overall impression of the biological, psychological and social factors impacting on the individual's distress and disability. So when we met Diane in clinic, for example, we had already gathered a lot of information about the way she was affected by persistent pain. Diane's psychometric tests revealed that she had high levels of kinesiophobia, informed by her own theories of why she had persistent pain: she believed that her spine was crumbling, and that the MRI scan of her lumbar spine showed defects in the discs. Avoiding movement was therefore important in order to halt the progression of the crumbling. Diane had become severely disabled due to this belief system and she scored very high on the disability questionnaire, spending much of her time in bed and experiencing difficulties with every aspect of daily life as indicated in her Brief Pain Inventory. Diane also catastrophized to a high degree, particularly with regards to ruminating about pain on a constant basis, and she had high levels of cognitive anxiety and pain-related fear. She scored in the moderately severe range for depression and in the severe range with regards to anxiety.

Diane's questionnaire also revealed to us that she had a pre-existing history of depression and anxiety and was a heavy smoker. There had been a significant change in the family dynamics due to the impact of her pain experience; she reported that her husband and mother had taken over most of the household chores and that she was depressed and anxious over losing her role as mother and caregiver to her children. The loss of her job had resulted in financial difficulties and the whole family had to change because she could no longer fulfil her previous roles. She had a very angry son who could remember her prior to the development of chronic pain and felt the loss of his mother. Her questionnaire revealed that she was looking for a quick fix for the management of her symptoms.

During the consultation Diane held her breath when attempting any movement; she would brace herself and groan when reaching for her handbag. Her husband answered a lot of questions for her – she asked him to and looked to him for answers but then got angry when he appeared to do most of the talking. Diane raged at the multiple injections into her spine that she had undergone without any benefit. She was angry that nobody had ever explained to her why she had developed persistent pain and she was also angry that it had taken years for her to have an MRI scan of her spine – she believed an earlier scan would have resulted in an operation to fix her back but that her spine was now beyond repair. Diane therefore presented as a patient at the more extreme end of the spectrum of individuals that we see.

*

The completed questionnaires returned by the patient to the pain centre are assessed by our physiotherapists who triage the referrals into various clinics. Patients who have been sent to the pain service for very specific management around medication or injections, or those who have significant medical co-morbidities and who are elderly, are often triaged to a 'doctor-only' clinic. The reason for this is that they may require some rehabilitation input but their concurrent medical problems, such as heart disease or respiratory disease, potentially preclude them from the physical reconditioning which is a component of the rehabilitation within the pain service.

Patients who score high on the depression inventory are triaged to a clinic slot called 'doctor-only complex'. These complex patients require more time during the assessment and it is often necessary to unpack their previous interactions with other clinicians. A patient like Diane, for example, would require a thorough and detailed explanation about the nature of chronic pain. I spent a long time with Diane talking about acute pain versus chronic pain and essentially explaining to her how the human body works. I often talk a lot in these sessions about the pain alarm system and use multiple analogies to try to convey the message that the ongoing pain is due to dysfunction of the pain alarm system rather than being due to ongoing damage. This message is very difficult for patients to receive and is often met with anger and disbelief. The anger is around having a condition which does not promise a cure and also at why it has taken so long for somebody to explain the condition to them. There is disbelief at why other doctors have offered treatments which, based on the theory I've proposed, clearly had no hope of helping their pain.

Much of the consultation is spent discussing the nature of chronic pain. I will explain very briefly the therapies that we offer within the pain service and the strategies that we employ to help people cope with chronic pain, but at that point patients are often not willing to hear what the future holds for them. The belief tends to persist that an injection, a medication or an operation is the only therapy that has any validity – this is often the case even where patients have tried this approach and it has failed. When we start talking about pacing day-to-day activities, or mindfulness, or solving problems in a more realistic way, patients become impatient.

Where the physiotherapists who triage the referrals feel that the patient may be suitable for rehabilitation – for example patients who present with musculoskeletal pain such as lower-back pain or other widespread chronic pain conditions such as fibromyalgia syndrome, but who have lower levels of psychological distress – they are placed into a clinic where the doctor assesses the patient with a physiotherapist. The physiotherapist in many ways does the same assessment that the doctor does, but the power of this consultation is the interaction between the doctor, the physiotherapist and the patient. Unfortunately, these consultations can be fraught, particularly when the physiotherapist is introduced. Patients who have had persistent pain for a long time have often already stopped at the train station marked physiotherapy. Their visit to that city has often been filled with disappointment and unmet expectations. There is no way that you can exercise, massage or manipulate your way out of chronic pain, and often patients will in fact experience flare-ups of pain due to hands-on physiotherapy, and this experience may prejudice them against the entire world of physiotherapy. They therefore view our physiotherapists with suspicion and frustration, and it is to the physiotherapist's credit that patients who are initially quite averse to physiotherapy leave feeling very reassured. The pain-management physiotherapists are experts at explaining to patients how changes in the way that activities are performed can lead to an improvement in their quality of life. Patients triaged in this clinic are often not as highly distressed as Diane and are therefore more receptive to receiving the message that their condition is not curable but can be managed.

The triage process also identifies patients who can be seen by a physiotherapist working independently. These patients usually do not require any medical input, and if after the initial assessment they have any questions that the physiotherapist is unable to answer, or if the physiotherapist feels that the answers the patient requires need to come from a doctor, then they will see one of the pain consultants. Whilst in my view the mainstay of pain management falls within the remit of psychologists and physiotherapists, the reality of the medical industrial complex is that the word of a doctor still carries more weight with many patients.

The doctor-only complex clinics are the hardest emotionally. Usually a thorough reading of the triage questionnaire provides you with an idea of how much anger, disappointment and resistance to change you may be faced with. The free-text answer to the question about expectations from the pain service is often at the crux of the interaction, as well as ideas about chronic pain which usually relate back to what the patient has understood from previous clinicians, for example that their back pain is due to their spine crumbling. The most challenging consultations are those where the patient has been referred to the pain centre by a clinician who has made promises to the patient that they will have an intervention that is not appropriate.

Over the years my approach to the management of patients with chronic pain has changed. There was a time when I believed that everybody could be saved by the miracle of pain management and that if I was skilful enough in communicating information about chronic pain and how this condition could be dealt with then everybody would be able to lead amazing and productive lives. I suppose this is no different from the enthusiasm which people who understand the benefits of healthy eating and physical exercise try to communicate to their clients. I have, however, come to accept both in the arena of pain management and in medical education (as well as in every relationship that I have had) that all one can do is your best, trying to be as creative as possible in communicating information, and employing feedback from the people you're trying to serve to inform your practice.

*

The consultation starts with me walking out to the waiting room to receive somebody. Often the assessment will begin at that point in terms of noticing who they are with and how they are walking. You can tell a lot about somebody simply by the way that they walk and carry themselves. I usually invite partners in but sometimes the patient tells the person who has accompanied them to remain outside, and the reason for this often becomes clear over the course of the next hour. If I am with a physiotherapist, they spend some time explaining the role of physiotherapy in pain management. Then I usually try to summarize the questionnaire that I have received from the patient. I have found that being able to recite details about their lives and the answers they have given to the questionnaires gives them some comfort in terms of feeling understood and listened to. Not being listened to by healthcare professionals, particularly doctors, is often the major complaint of patients who attend the pain clinic. Being able to recount intimate details of their understanding of pain builds an automatic rapport.

I usually have to explain what our pain clinic offers, particularly to patients who have been to other pain clinics before. I did this with Diane. I started with an explanation of chronic pain and how our belief is that the pain is due to changes within the nerves and how they function rather than due to ongoing damage. I talked about the fact that patients who have had limbs amputated continue to experience pain even though the limb is no longer there and therefore cannot possibly be damaged, but that the pain is still experienced because the nerve which used to go down to the limb is still present and travels from the stump to the brain. I explained that it was very difficult for us to stop these abnormal sensations and that our pain clinic worked with people in order to try to get them to live productively with the constant presence of pain rather than trying to attempt to cure the condition. I adopt this approach sometimes with patients who have a long history of persistent pain and who have had multiple negative interactions with clinicians. Setting out your stall immediately at least gives the person the option of walking out or alternatively, and hopefully, allows them to manage their expectations at the outset with regards to what they can anticipate from this pain clinic.

The history taken during the consultation is largely an attempt to understand the person and how they and their loved ones live with chronic pain. By the time they reach the pain clinic most serious conditions have been excluded. There are many pain consultants who argue that they are not diagnosticians and that they cannot be held responsible for missing pathology. A couple of times in the last decade I have picked up cancers of the spine, but in these cases the patients presented with pain and risk factors that made it patently obvious that there was something else going on. Most patients have had a thorough set of investigations done prior to coming to the pain centre and it is usually very clear that we are dealing with a chronic non-malignant pain condition. This does not stop patients feeling that they need further investigations and much of the to-ing and fro-ing between the rehabilitation team and the medical consultant in the pain service revolves around the desire of patients to check that nothing has been missed.

I ask patients about their pain and focus on how pain impacts on their ability to perform the basic activities of daily living, including washing and dressing, as well as making breakfast, lunch and dinner, and sleeping. I ask about how they spend their days. Those patients who are working (and they are often in the minority) are asked about how their employer interacts with them in terms of their chronic pain condition and whether adaptations and allowances have been made in the workplace. Most patients spend a lot of time watching TV, smoking cigarettes and staring into space. This presents a challenging scenario with regards to rehabilitation because in many ways having chronic pain has become the sufferer's occupation and any attempt at rehabilitation threatens the homeostasis that has now evolved within the household.

Sleep is significantly disrupted by persistent pain and we spend a lot of time focused on how the person sleeps and whether they nap during the day. Fatigue is intimately associated with chronic pain, since the brain areas which sub-serve these functions are both located in the same region. Chronic fatigue syndrome and chronic widespread pain often coexist, each feeding off the other. We ask patients about their mood and anxiety and enquire specifically about acts of self-harm. We discuss medications and how useful these are in the management of persistent pain and try to identify patterns of behaviour which point to addiction or dependence. We do ask about previous life events, but I try not to delve too deeply, because once you start scratching the surface with chronic pain patients there are issues which arise that I am not qualified to contain. A history of sexual abuse is not uncommon, as is domestic violence and difficult social circumstances. The question which is of fundamental importance and sets the tone for further engagement in the service, however, is the patient's understanding of why their pain has persisted. Patients will tell you stories that involve surgeons having told them: 'I would operate but the operation would probably kill you'; 'Your discs are crumbling and there is nothing we can do because the hospital will not pay for disc replacement surgery'; 'I could help you but you're too fat'. Patients may have been told that the pain is all in their head and often when I explain the nature of chronic pain as not being due to disease or injury this is interpreted by the patient as it being dismissed as imaginary pain. This belief may have been reinforced by some of the clinicians whom they have seen who refer to such concepts as psychosomatic pain or psychologically mediated pain. Our psychologists have had to write a leaflet explaining the role of clinical psychology in the management of pain and explaining pain to patients has become a significant industry.

Patients like Diane are not going to be helped by further interventions. The diagnosis I made at the end of our consultation was that she had non-specific lower-back pain with pain-associated reduction in physical functioning, and the psychological impact in terms of anxiety and depression of having a persistent pain condition was impairing her ability to function. Biologically Diane's pain was maintained by changes in the pain alarm system but there was no evidence that she suffered with compression of her nerves in the spine based on the MRI scan. There was therefore no surgical cause or remedy for her pain.

Diane's assessment described the biopsychosocial formulation of her chronic pain condition. Targets for her rehabilitation included education around the management of pain as well as learning adaptive coping strategies from our psychologists. The aim was to reduce the fear Diane experienced by helping her to understand that her condition was not due to ongoing damage; this would then allow her to gradually start increasing her levels of activity in a paced manner under the guidance of our physiotherapists. From the medical point of view, her use of opioids was destructive in that it affected her ability to think, and I suspected that at some point she had become addicted to the opioids because despite them not providing any benefit she continued to use them. We would therefore have to address opioid reduction as part of her overall pain management strategy. Diane presented with clear targets for successful participation in rehabilitation, but these were ultimately our goals and our assessment and at the end of the day it would be down to whether Diane chose to continue living in the way that she currently was or engaged with our service in order to make changes.

There was a time when I would refer somebody like Diane to one of our psychologists immediately because of the score on her depression psychometric. A score above a certain threshold triages an immediate referral to psychology as the next point of contact within the service, but this number is fairly arbitrary and there are some patients whose low mood is perfectly understandable in the context of their pain and its impact on their function, and when you explain chronic pain to them they appear to accept the explanation and are able to see the sense in what you are offering. In these instances, I will exercise my discretion and refer them on to the physiotherapy team. My practice now is not to refer somebody like Diane immediately to psychology because inevitably patients who do not accept or understand the chronic pain paradigm that we operate within will not attend what is a very costly appointment to provide.

I offer patients the opportunity to come back and see me if they have further questions about the nature of chronic pain – particularly with regards to whether they have structural problems or the need for further medical investigation – or they can opt in to rehabilitation and see a physiotherapist or psychologist. Our physiotherapists have devised an opt-in system because of the high level of non-attenders they have at their clinics. The hope is that there will be fewer patients who do not attend because the act of opting in implies a willingness to change.

*

I see new patients on a Wednesday morning. In order to prepare for the clinic, I spend an hour in the gym from 6.00 a.m. I also spend time in the sauna and steam room to mentally prepare for the next four hours, as I have realized that there is the potential for a significant amount of drama during that time. When I talk to people who work in difficult clinical environments, I often use Karpman's Drama Triangle as a model for being aware of the potential for conflict in any given situation. Karpman used a triangle to map the various roles people play within drama-intense interactions, defining three roles present in any conflict situation: persecutor, rescuer and victim. The victim's stance is essentially that of feeling oppressed, helpless and hopeless, as well as powerless and ashamed, with an inability to make decisions. Patients who present with persistent pain, by the very nature of the condition, often adopt this role or have developed these strategies over time. When a patient who is playing the victim role presents in clinic, they often position the doctor as either the rescuer or the persecutor.

The rescuer feels guilty if he or she doesn't go to the rescue, which is often what leads to patients having inappropriate investigations or interventions; playing the role of the rescuer allows the pressure to be taken off them by focusing their energies on doing something for the victim. The persecutor, on the other hand, insists that the problem is all the victim's fault and is blaming, critical, authoritative, rigid and superior. Patients who have had interventions fail often switch to the persecutor role because of promises made by the clinician which have not come to fruition. The clinician then ends up becoming the victim and so the drama continues.

When I am in clinic, I try to almost exist outside myself at times in order to observe the interaction at a distance. I try to monitor how I'm feeling at any point and whenever I feel that I have adopted any of these roles I pause and analyse the situation. I think that most doctors struggle with not ending up being a rescuer. Many people who go into healthcare roles do so because they enjoy the pay-off that comes from being able to focus on helping others as opposed to becoming more integrated people themselves. I sometimes wonder if the desire to be an interventional pain doctor stems from the self-esteem boost that comes from providing therapies – even though they only work occasionally, this is often enough. I have noticed lately that this behaviour manifests as doctors posting patient testimonials about the treatments they have provided on social media platforms. Unfortunately, this does tend to lead to co-dependency – for example, the giving of repeated injections encourages the patient to adopt a passive approach to their pain management, aided and abetted by a well-meaning physician or one who benefits financially or psychologically from performing repeat procedures.

The corollary of Karpman's Triangle is the Winner's Triangle by Acey Choy, published in 1990. Choy proposed a reimagining of the three states of rescuer, victim and persecutor. Anyone feeling like a victim should think more in terms of being vulnerable and caring, and should be encouraged to accept this and become more self-aware; anybody cast as a persecutor should adopt a positive and assertive role and should be encouraged to ask the 'victim' what it is that they want; the rescuer should be encouraged to show concern and care but not overreach and problem-solve for others. As a doctor, understanding which role you are being cast in within a clinical context and changing to the corresponding Winner's position makes for a more productive clinic. Burnout is an ever-present threat to doctors who work in these dramatic situations that are filled with potential conflict, and understanding your role and your own psychological vulnerability is the only way to ensure that you are able to provide good care. The alternative to the above is the tuckshop in the corner of our coffee room which is stocked by one of the nurses. I always know when one of the psychologists has had a difficult morning because of their very fast walk to the corner where the chocolate is kept.

*

Having come in and spoken to me, Diane rang our number the following day. She told the receptionist, Julie, that she had read the patient information leaflet and whilst she was not 100 per cent convinced by the explanation that I gave her, she felt that she had run out of options with regards to her pain and was keen to improve her quality of life. Julie then triggered the referral letter to our pain management psychologist, which I composed alongside the letter to Diane's GP.

The psychologists usually see patients for around ninety minutes. Their assessments are in-depth and venture into areas of previous and current psychological functioning as well as psychosocial factors which impact on the development and maintenance of chronic pain. Individuals are usually seen by themselves initially and then their partners are brought in towards the end of the appointment to further add to the depth of the assessment. The psychologist will analyse in more detail the scores on the psychometric tests which focus on depression, anxiety and catastrophizing along with the patient's daily routine, current sleep hygiene and the impact of pain on their social lives. The psychologist will also delve into the early life of the individual and psychological injuries sustained during their formative years, which may impact on their ability to cope. Previous reactions to grief and the ability to surmount these reactions are also discussed. Ultimately the aim of the psychology assessment is to identify any barriers to participation in rehabilitation, as a result of which the patient may be referred to the pain physician for further discussions to try to facilitate reassurance or action appropriate investigations. The patient's suitability for group work versus individual work is assessed, as well as identifying what the person's goals are with regards to rehabilitation.

After the psychology assessment Diane was referred to the physiotherapy team who assessed her current level of functioning and whether she would fit into the context of a pain management programme. Her ability to self-care and whether she would be able to turn up daily for a programme was assessed together with her beliefs and understanding about pain and her perception and experience of the safety of movement.

The fundamental underpinning of pain management psychology is the idea that excitatory pain pathways which send a barrage of information about harm or potential harm become active and the inhibitory pain pathways that attempt to quell this information are compromised in the presence of anxiety, depression, threat and catastrophic thoughts about pain. When patients learn to regain control over these emotive responses using methods such as cognitive behavioural therapy and mindfulness, they are then potentially able to activate inhibitory pain pathways and regain some control over the intrusiveness of pain despite not abolishing it. In the future it may be that rather than aiming to use psychological methods to teach people to accept pain and to improve their function, behavioural techniques may be specific and targeted enough to reduce the actual experience of pain. According to the authors of a paper entitled 'When pain gets stuck: the evolution of pain chronification and treatment resistance', there is a need for a closer relationship between the neurobiology of pain and attempts to influence behaviour. 'Hurt does not mean harm' is the basis for any psychology-based pain management therapy. Overturning the idea that chronic pain is an alarm to avoid harm sits at the centre of rehabilitation, and until a patient accepts that persistent pain is not a harbinger of further injury, fixed pain behaviours such as fear-induced avoidance cannot be unlocked. According to the authors of 'When pain gets stuck', the next generation of psychology-based medicine will move away from encouraging this acceptance of pain and will instead seek to alter that inevitability.

Current pain management rehabilitation, however, focuses on improvement in function, psychological well-being and quality of life, despite the ongoing presence of persistent pain. We do not yet have reliable techniques to actually reduce pain through psychology-based interventions and any attempt to link pain directly to a patient's psychology can lead to failure and reinforce the idea that the pain is all in the patient's head. The rehabilitation team employ a 'five systems' model to help patients learn to manage persistent pain effectively. The five systems consider the **trigger situation** and how it interacts with the individual's **thoughts** (perceptions and predictions of the situation which are often silent conversations that an individual has with him- or herself), **emotions**, **behaviour** and **physiology** (including bodily reactions which are felt internally by the individual and not externally observed).

One of our psychologists, when he teaches this model and how it applies to pain medicine, uses the example of a man who is waiting to go on his first date. The environmental trigger is that of waiting for a first date. His thoughts might revolve around potential embarrassments, such as saying the wrong thing or wearing the wrong clothes. Emotionally he then feels anxious. Physiologically he might experience an increase in muscle tension with an increase in heart rate, sweating and fast and shallow breathing. His behaviour during the date may then be inhibited or alternatively he might decide to abandon the endeavour altogether. If he abandons going on the date, he feels relieved as he leaves but he becomes disabled in an important aspect of life. His dating 'self-efficacy' (self-efficacy is defined as a personal conviction that one can successfully execute a course of action to produce a desired outcome in a situation) remains low and he is likely to continue to remain anxious in similar situations (he is also likely to remain single). He is therefore at risk of continued avoidant coping and ongoing impairment in his ability to date.

A similar example applied to somebody with chronic pain could have putting their socks on as the trigger. The person may think, 'If I bend over I'm going to prolapse my disc again and end up paralysed.' They then experience fear and panic at the thought of performing the activity, causing an increase in muscle tension and pain; the behavioural response is one of breath-holding because of the feelings of fear and panic, they avoid bending over and their partner puts their socks on for them. There is obvious relief at not having to bend and suffer the imagined risk of a disc prolapse and the socks are on their feet (mission accomplished), however they have become disabled in an important aspect of their self-care function and tomorrow morning will feel anxious again about dressing. The action of the partner has resulted in a disabling and overprotective pattern being reinforced. The person with pain has also not moved their back in a normal manner and this contributes to further deconditioning. Fear of falling and flare-ups of pain as well as self-consciousness about pain behaviours and loss of social confidence and work are also environmental triggers.

Trigger situations result in feelings of anxiety and fear leading to avoidant behaviour. Avoidant behaviour results in short-term relief of anxiety but in the long term there is no opportunity to build confidence and so individuals continue to experience anxiety about situations that occur as part of everyday life. The aim of rehabilitation is to increase tolerance to trigger situations, and psychology-based pain management utilizes the concept of behavioural activation which encourages the individual to use *approaching* rather than *avoiding* behaviours and to become active despite their negative feelings or lack of motivation. Repeated practice in the same situation results in progressively reduced anxiety with each exposure. The aim of pain management rehabilitation is to help the individual to break down an anxiety-provoking activity into a series of steps. The initial steps up a ladder are difficult but once the patient builds up confidence that the situation can be tolerated then the higher steps become easier to navigate. Situations therefore become less anxiety-provoking.

Behavioural activation uses the principles of operant conditioning or associative learning, reworking a patient's association between an action and the likely consequences, encouraging depressed people to reconnect with their environment and facilitate positive reinforcement. The aim for Diane was to carry out regular and manageable as well as meaningful activities that are an important part of day-to-day function, leading to greater enjoyment and satisfaction and helping her to recover some of her previous feelings of self-worth.

The important point to note, and this is the most difficult one for patients to accept when you meet them in the clinic, is that rehabilitation and behavioural activation take place in the absence of any meaningful reduction in pain. We are conditioned to believe that rehabilitation should only take place once the pain has stopped, particularly when it comes to acute injuries. Interestingly, even with performance athletes and acute injury, we have moved away from the idea of waiting for a reduction in pain before rehabilitation takes place. It is now known that recovery can be enhanced if movement takes place early; active recovery is now undertaken by athletes following games and might include yoga rather than rest. Medically, this technique is used in the context of patients who have had surgery for cancer, where early mobilization has been shown to reduce complications.

Diane had expressed some concerns in her initial appointment about her spine and its structural stability. Successive appointments with the physiotherapist and psychologist as well as detailed explanations about the way the spine functions had reassured her to a degree and she was now willing to start thinking about exercise. Earlier in her life with persistent pain she had experienced good days and bad days with regards to the intensity of her pain, and this had led her to do too much on a good day. She said that she would rush about and do all the activities which she was prevented from doing on a bad day. Unfortunately, she would then experience an increase in pain on successive days and eventually stopped having good days and behaving in this way. She was therefore used to trying to do activities despite the presence of pain. Whilst Diane was spending an excessive amount of time at home, she was not spending it in bed. Spending time in bed and not being able to self-care are potential barriers to engaging in a pain management programme.

*

Diane was listed for our intensive programme which runs for fifteen sessions, from 9.30 a.m. to 4.30 p.m., Monday to Friday, over a three-week period, and patients are then followed up at one, three and six months. Residential places are available for patients who travel from far away. Patients listed for intensive programmes are less functional and have higher levels of distress and fear-induced avoidance than is the case for those attending the standard pain management programme, which runs for eight sessions over four weeks with patients attending twice a week. The standard programme is more suitable for local patients who have greater functionality and lower levels of distress and they are also more likely to be in work.

At the first session of the programme, I often talk about the limitations of the biomedical model and how restricted we are in terms of our science and understanding of many conditions, including persistent pain. We spend some time talking about the value of imaging in the form of X-rays and MRI scans. I talk about how doctors are trained and why patients have often come across doctors with different theories of why they have pain. I try to communicate to patients that what is needed most for patients who suffer with pain, and across the general population, is a reorientation with regards to the medical profession and the treatments that we offer. I encourage patients to question their doctors when it comes to any diagnosis or treatment, and to ask about risks and benefits. Most patients, particularly in the UK, have a very passive approach to their healthcare; doctors are still perceived to be the final arbiters of decision-making in a determinedly paternalistic system. My talk lasts about half an hour, after which the psychologist and physiotherapist set out their stalls.

The aims of the psychologists are to help patients move from the medical model of pain to the biopsychosocial model of pain and disability and to educate them about the physiological effects of pain. Psychologists help patients to build up their self-management skills and to reduce their reliance on healthcare professionals. Barriers to progress are addressed and positive lifestyle changes are encouraged. Psychologists focus on the stress response and its impact on muscular activity. We use a picture of an EMG (electro-myography) recording which shows the electrical response of muscles in patients with chronic lower-back pain and contrasts it with the electrical response of people without pain. In individuals who do not have chronic pain there is a lack of electrical activity when the person is stationary and bending forward, whereas in patients who have persistent pain the EMG shows ongoing electrical activity through-out the cycle of movement. We use this to indicate how techniques such as relaxation training and diaphragmatic breathing can calm down these hyperirritable muscles and therefore reduce the physiological response to pain.

The psychologist will also teach the patients the cogni-tive behavioural therapy skills which I mentioned above, including a behavioural approach to the management of environmental triggers, as well as focusing on sleep hygiene and sexual relationships. Chronic pain inevitably spikes due to psychosocial stressors, and so adaptive ways of dealing with these flare-ups are taught. The partners are invited to a session in an attempt to try to help them understand what living with chronic pain is like and what constitutes helpful and unhelpful behaviours in those living with the patient.

The physiotherapy sessions teach patients how to split activities into manageable portions and to gradually increase levels of activity through pacing. Patients are taught the importance of posture and biomechanics and are actively engaged in exercises which include stretching and strengthening as well as aerobic and pool sessions.

I will see the patients on both the intensive and standard programmes again during the course, at which point we have a longer discussion about the role of medications and interventions. Much of what I tell patients is recorded in this book. I will often ask patients to tell me how much pain relief they have obtained from medications and consistently the answer comes up as 30 per cent, which is congruent with the scientific literature. Despite this, many patients who have had negative experiences with medications are still married to the idea of taking a drug and cannot escape the mindset of seeking a pharmacological solution to their pain.

We talk about interventional pain therapies, including injections and surgery, and I explain how complex the nervous system is and how merely changing how a structure within the body looks by performing an operation – as in the case of a knee replacement or the decompression of a nerve – does not necessarily change how the nerves which supply the structure function. A patient with a beautifully decompressed spinal nerve may continue to experience their preoperative pain – sometimes more severely.

Even if a knee replacement is completely technically successful and you have changed the architecture of the knee, the nerves which supply the knee were already exhibiting aberrant function and therefore fail to settle regardless of how beautiful the post-operative X-ray of the knee looks to the orthopaedic surgeon. The concept that the brain constantly monitors the body for signs of deviation rather than being a passive recipient of information may explain why joint replacement sometimes does not work, as changing the biological knee for an artificial one does not change the brain's perception of what is happening to the joint. Risk factors for continuing to experience knee pain following a technically successful replacement include catastrophizing, depression and the presence of chronic pain at another site. All knees change as we grow older, just as faces change and wrinkles appear. The changes in the knee, however, do not relate proportionately and precisely to the pain experienced and it may be that the deformation of the knee due to being overweight, for example, is what the brain responds to and which causes pain; what is needed to reduce the knee pain is in fact weight loss and strengthening the muscles which support the joint.

I find these sessions enjoyable and personally educational. I have changed my style of delivery over the years, moving from death by PowerPoint to simply having a conversation with people. I spend less time talking and more time listening. It is crucial to establish at the beginning of the programme the patients' ideas, concerns and expectations with regards to pain management from a medical point of view, or they will fail to engage.

The patients tend to be both hopeful and anxious; there is a real desire in the room for change and improvement. As a medic you only get a glimpse into the transformative power of a pain management programme; the psychologists and physiotherapists are the ones who accompany patients along the journey to improved function. This includes social function, and there is often an outing to the local swimming pool or ten-pin bowling. Patients choose what activities they would like to do and for many of them this is the first time in forever that they have done anything approaching recreational activity.

I often see the patients as they check-in each morning when they are on a programme. I always leave my clinic door open (when I'm not seeing patients) and watch them walk by, and over a three-week period there is a noticeable difference in the way that they walk; I notice a reduction in pain behaviours and a faster pace of activity. It is very compelling to appreciate that we have not given these patients an injection or a drug – the patient simply realizes that by changing their thoughts about pain and changing their behaviour they can transform their ability to function.

The final interaction I have with the patients on the programme is an individual review where we discuss their current medication and hopefully have a discussion around reducing it. From time to time we do have programme attendees who ask us about new drugs (cannabis oil has become the bane of my life) or interventions and it becomes obvious during the consultation that the person has not really bought into the ethos of the programme. The reality is that this person will continue to seek a cure for a condition which they are in denial about. Then there are those who make progress but fear what will happen when they leave the comfort and support of a group. Patients from a programme often keep in contact with one another, and a card usually appears in our coffee room from the participants to the team who have delivered the pain management programme. I think it is easy for a doctor to become cynical about chronic pain management and the biobehavioural approach because we only tend to see those patients who fail to progress, but for our psychologists and physiotherapists, delivering pain management programmes is a rewarding activity.

*

Diane completed the programme. Afterwards, she reflected that a year ago she had a rain cloud hanging over her head which was filled with negative thoughts; she felt sleepy, tired and lethargic all the time and had no interest in any activities. She never left the house alone. Diane felt over-weight, miserable and was tearful for much of the time. Her activities involved Internet shopping at ungodly hours, and she had difficulty walking, cooking and climbing stairs. Three months after the programme she felt happy and had lost weight (and gained it back, but was attending Slimming

World). She had a positive, can-do attitude and had regained her interest in life. She was able to leave the house and enjoy social occasions and activity. Six months later, she writes that she is happy with life and has lost weight again. She feels able to make decisions about the future and is now considering possibly working and is even more active.

Diane's story shows the potential positive effect of pain management programmes, but unfortunately these programmes are not a panacea. Chronic pain is exactly that – it is chronic and unrelenting and human beings struggle with diseases that require active self-management and a life-long commitment to wellness. The difference in outcome between two patients is often not medical input but the person's commitment to managing their condition. In one UK interdisciplinary pain management centre, tracking patients on a residential pain management programme, clinically significant gains on pain and psychological measures were achieved by 19 to 55 per cent of the patients at post-treatment and 17 to 44 per cent at a nine-month follow-up assessment. This means that no improvement in pain or psychological measures may occur in 45 to 71 per cent immediately post-treatment and 56 to 83 per cent of patients at follow-up.

There are no studies looking at the long-term outcomes of patients who have participated in a pain management programme. The detractors of this form of therapy (usually doctors involved in interventional pain therapies) cite the lack of long-term follow-up as a reason for persisting in trying to achieve pain *relief*. As with all things in life the truth lies somewhere in between. Unfortunately, both camps tend to be polarized in their points of view and stick religiously to the fundamental tenets of their paradigms.

I feel more at peace these days when I sit in my new patient pain clinic. I am less the George Michael of 'Club Tropicana', 'Young Guns' and 'Careless Whisper' and more 'Faith', 'Older' and 'Heal the Pain'. This peace and acceptance of my role has come after a long time. When I started as a consultant, I believed that I could save everybody by selling them interdisciplinary rehabilitation. I felt that I could bring everybody back to psychological health and back to the light. I thought that I could get everybody with chronic pain to successfully pace their activities, to engage with and understand pain, and overcome it with newly discovered resilience. I was a true and indiscriminate believer. I would often get quite cross with one of our physiotherapists who has been around for a while because she didn't seem that hopeful about most patients. In retrospect I realize that her experience over the years has given her a very clear sense of those patients who will engage with pain management and those who will not. The reality of a pain clinic is that I think we actually help about 10 per cent of people who suffer with chronic pain and who present to our clinic to move forward with their lives, according to our outcome measures, whilst the rest find some way to live with their condition, usually in a way that we would consider not adaptive or contributing to society, but which works in their world.

Chronic pain cannot as yet be cured. Neither can diabetes mellitus or high blood pressure for that matter. The aim is to focus on reducing the distress and disability of a life of persistent pain. Multimodal pain management – collaborative and integrated use of needles, narcotics and knives along with words and understanding – probably represents the kindest, most effective and least harmful approach to the management of the disease that is chronic pain. Interdisciplinary collaboration – psychologists working with doctors working with physiotherapists working with occupational therapists and nurses – where the biological and the behavioural are addressed by a team operating with the same philosophy, seems to be the best way to deliver this care.

Torpedo fish

'I feel as if someone is putting out a thousand cigarettes on my leg. Sometimes it feels as if skittles are being thrown on to my leg and no matter which part of the outer side of my leg I touch the sensation is always felt somewhere else.'

'I don't know if you have children, Doctor, but imagine that you wake up in the middle of the night to go to the toilet and you have to walk down a dark passage in your home to get there. You had a long week and probably too much to drink the night before. You didn't get the promotion that you went for and so probably won't be able to afford the holiday you promised the children. One of your children has left their Lego in the middle of the corridor and you step on it. The awkwardness of the shape of the Lego as it bruises your foot and the horrible numbing, electric-like pain is how my leg feels all the time. I feel as if hundreds of Lego pieces are being pressed into my leg all the time and the disappointment of the children and the lack of promotion and the feeling of weariness never stops.'

'The burning never stops. Sometimes during the day I can forget it for a little while, but at night when everything is quiet it returns. I toss and turn, and I cannot bear to have the bedclothes touch my legs. I know it's my fault, I know I should have managed my diabetes better.'

The testimonies above are from patients who have neuropathic pain, which I have touched upon in some of the preceding chapters. Neuropathic pain is pain due to disease or injury of the system that registers and reports sensation (nerves) and affects 6 to 8 per cent of the adult population. When you have non-specific lower-back pain – non-specific in the sense that the pain is not linked to a fracture of the spine or compression of a nerve or inflammation of the joints – the pain tends to trouble you in a predictable pattern, perhaps when you sit or stand for long periods or lift something heavy. Patients can usually therefore adopt strategies to minimize pain. They generally tend to be okay when pacing gentle activities such as watching TV, and pain only becomes a problem when they exceed their usual activity levels. For patients with nerve damage the experiences of pain are materially different: pain is unpredictable and consists of odd sensations which doctors refer to as positive and negative symptoms. A positive symptom would be something like an abnormal feeling or sensation called a paraesthesia, which when experienced as unpleasant is called dysaesthesia. Patients also experience tingling and burning as described in the testimonies above. Negative symptoms are those of numbness or loss of sensation, in which patients experience the disturbing paradox of feeling pain even though the area affected is numb.

Nerve pain tends to affect a specific body area because nerves give sensation and power to certain areas. Where the peripheral nervous system is affected (from traumatic nerve damage or sciatica or diseases such as diabetes) this usually involves the legs or arms. The peripheral nervous system consists of all the nerves which radiate from the spinal cord and from the brain, but does not include the brain or spinal cord themselves, which are referred to as the central nervous system. Central nervous system disorders such as multiple sclerosis and strokes, it could be argued, cause even worse symptoms and patients may have severe debilitating neuropathic pain which is also accompanied by deficits in the function of their muscles (with associated spasticity and musculoskeletal pain) and often their bladders and bowels don't work properly.

Nerve pain can mimic other non-neuropathic pain conditions and we therefore take great care when diagnosing this problem. The patient must have a disease or injury of a nerve which can logically explain their symptoms. They then must have both positive and negative symptoms and signs (things doctors look for on examination) such as decreased sensation to cotton wool or a pinprick, or increased pain and sensitivity within the distribution of that nerve territory. If we are still not sure, nerve conduction studies can be ordered to confirm the diagnosis. These tests consist of placing needles into muscles and measuring the electrical activity along the nerve to assess if the nerve has been injured. It is, however, possible to have nerve damage but still register normal electrical results, as the tests are simply not sensitive enough to detect the damage that has occurred in some cases.

The most common neuropathic pain conditions that I see in clinic are patients who have had prolapsed discs which have damaged the nerves as they leave the spinal canal either through a chemical irritation or direct compression. We still don't know what the precise evolution of long-term pain from a prolapsed disc is, and there are patients with disc prolapses identified on MRI scans who never develop persistent nerve pain. We also see patients who have nerve pain from diabetes, where chronic high blood sugars have destroyed the blood vessels supplying oxygen to nerves which then die and regenerate haphazardly, resulting in pain in the arms and legs – often referred to as a glove and stocking distribution of pain. Most neuropathic patients are resigned to a life on antidepressant medication and anti-epileptic medication to treat their nerve pain, and I have already described how poor these medications are in terms of relieving pain. At best they may get 30 to 50 per cent pain relief, often at the cost of impairing their ability to concentrate and function; they are transformed into the walking dead, shadows of their former selves. Inevitably, due to their complaints of persistent pain and distress when they see their GP, they are started on opioids which escalate over time. This opioid haze does not improve their experience of pain but will further affect their ability to function.

Of all the patients I see in the pain clinic, the patients who suffer with neuropathic pain are probably the ones who have the best chance of finding a biomedical solution for alleviating their pain. Most of the patients we see in pain clinics are treated with a combination of medication, pain management interventions (steroid and local anaesthetic injections or the burning of nerves) and pain management rehabilitation, which we discussed in the previous chapter. Peripheral neuropathic pain, however, is one of the few conditions where we can successfully modulate the abnormal information emanating from damaged nerves through electrical stimulation of areas of the spinal cord. When I talk to patients about this treatment, they look at me as if I was the reincarnation of Mary Shelley and the therapy I am offering straight from *Frankenstein*. The reason for this is because it involves modulating the nervous system with the application of an electrical current.

*

The first recorded effect of electricity on the human body dates back to 2500 BC. A picture illustrating a fisherman catching a Nile catfish and experiencing what looks like a painful shock was found painted on the wall of an Egyptian architect's tomb. Some 2000 years later, Aristotle mentions the effect of torpedo fish on other animals, and it was also recognized that the shock from the torpedo fish could be transmitted through a trident used to spear the animal. The numbing effect of the torpedo fish was used satirically to describe the effect of the conversation of Socrates on one of his pupils. It was a Roman physician called Scribonius Largus in the first century AD who first described the medical use of the torpedo fish when he cured Anteros, a court official of Emperor Tiberius, of his gout. He suggested that the patient should stand on the shore washed by the sea and he should stay this way until his whole foot and leg up to the knee was numb from being stung by the resident torpedo fish. Avicenna's text *The Canon of Medicine* recommends the use of torpedo fish to treat headaches, melancholy and for arresting epileptic seizures. The phenomenon of electricity was obviously not yet understood, and one Roman physician felt that the torpedo fish was releasing a venom.

Nearly 2000 years later, in the eighteenth century, Henry Cavendish constructed an artificial torpedo fish using devices for storing electric charge in a leather case resembling the size and shape of the fish. The flurry of experimentation into the phenomenon and subsequent increased understanding of the nature of electricity in this century resulted in an explosion of electricity-based devices used as medical therapies. Electrotherapy was put forward as a panacea not only for use by the medical profession but was also utilized by charlatans to exploit the vulnerable. It is probably this legacy which most influences patients' scepticism with regards to my proposal to use electricity to manage their pain.

The first electrical device designed specifically to manage pain was patented by Charles Willie Kent in 1919 and manufactured in Illinois; it was called the Electreat and was probably similar to a transcutaneous electrical nerve stimulator (TENS), which was developed much later and marketed as a treatment for every imaginable illness. The gate control theory by Melzack and Wall (see p. 44) was fundamental to the development of electrical pain management, as it proposed that pain perception is not (as Descartes had described) a line-labelled pathway which continues uninterrupted from the source of the injury to the brain but that the spinal cord acts as a gating mechanism which can be influenced in terms of pain perception. This paradigm shift in understanding pain opened the way for the development of electrical therapies to manage pain. Melzack and Wall proposed that the gate could be opened or closed depending on the balance between the stimulation of small and large nerves. When you step on a piece of Lego multiple behaviours which can influence the gate are activated: taking pressure off the foot, sitting down and swearing, and finally rubbing the foot all play a role in altering pain perception. The rubbing of the foot stimulates large fibres in the foot which compete with the smaller fibres transmitting the electrical stimulus encoding harm. The birth of the TENS machine was a direct result of this theory, in that by applying electrical stimulation to electrodes taped to the skin of the painful area the stimulation of the large fibres could be evoked. When I explain spinal cord stimulation to patients, they often immediately ask if it is similar to transcutaneous electrical nerve stimulation.

Implantable devices to stimulate nerves were initially placed near the peripheral nerves found superficially in the arms and legs. In 1967 Norman Shealy from the Western Reserve School of Medicine had the idea to stimulate the large nerve fibres as they gathered in the posterior columns of the spinal cord. Instead of stimulating these fibres through the skin peripherally, in his view they could be accessed directly where they bundled in the spinal cord. Theoretically this would enable a larger area of the body to be stimulated (more nerves servicing a larger area are found tightly packed in a small part of the spinal cord) than could be achieved by merely placing electrodes on the skin. The first model of the spinal cord stimulator involved an internally placed lead which entered the cerebrospinal fluid area and required an external power supply connected by a needle through the skin. Modern spinal cord stimulators are placed in the epidural space to avoid the complications which occur when the lead floats in the cerebrospinal fluid, and they do not require an external power supply. The first patient to have a stimulator implanted had cancer and it was used to successfully treat this person's cancer pain for four years.

The use of electricity to manage pain developed alongside the use of electricity to manage cardiovascular disease. The first spinal cord stimulators were essentially modified versions of the electrical devices used to treat hypertension. As devices developed initially, they consisted of an electrode with its antenna. The patient had a battery-operated power supply and controls which communicated with this antenna. By 1981 Medtronic, the company Shealy founded, produced a fully implantable device.

In the 1980s electrodes were introduced with multiple contacts which meant that different parts of the spinal cord could be stimulated, covering a wider pain area. In 2005 the first rechargeable battery for use in spinal cord stimulation was invented, which meant that batteries would need to be replaced less often and that more energy-demanding therapies could be used. Between 2005 and 2007 several landmark studies in spinal cord stimulation were carried out, which demonstrated that, for neuropathic pain due to lumbar spine problems, the therapy was more cost-effective and produced better pain relief than further surgery. The therapy has been approved by the National Institute for Health and Care Excellence (NICE) who issued formal guidance for the delivery of spinal cord stimulation in 2008 and reviewed it again in 2013, and it is supported globally by the International Neuromodulation Society.

Many studies have been done looking at whether the initial costs of the spinal cord stimulator are justified. At present, these devices cost north of £15,000–20,000, but it has been shown that this initial cost is worth it given the potential for avoiding repeat surgery or ongoing investigations, injections and drug therapy.

*

The apprehension that patients experience when I broach the subject of spinal cord stimulation is palpable. I often marvel at how patients will happily consent to the most horrific and invasive surgery, and will also often agree to take mind-altering substances, but the idea of inserting a device that is able to generate a current in their body (even though we are as people not shadows and dust but water and electricity) provokes immense distress. Electricity frightens people despite its silent presence in ensuring that our societies function – *Frankenstein*, homemade medical devices and the electric chair all play a role, I believe, in the acceptability (or otherwise) of electrical therapy. It is interesting, though, that patients will readily accept the use of a pacemaker. I suppose the reason for this difference is that without a pacemaker or an implantable cardiac defibrillator (which can deliver a shock should your heart stop) you will probably die. In the management of pain there is always the choice to live with your pain or not. As I often remind trainees, chronic pain doesn't kill anybody and therefore the acceptability of a therapy is always a careful assessment of risk and benefit, both on the part of the patient and the clinician. I remind myself constantly that any patient who comes into clinic, no matter how distressed, was living with their chronic pain the day before their appointment and will continue to live with chronic pain the day after, which makes me less likely to adopt the role of a rescuer in response to their presentation in the role of the victim.

Implanting a permanent device into a patient demands that the assessment process and the long-term care of the patient are handled by a neuromodulation team, formed from a subset of members from the wider pain service. The team must be able to assess the complexity of the patient and the therapy as well as the factors that will impact on the success of the treatment. First, patients are seen by myself or one of my colleagues who also implants these devices. Secondly, they are also evaluated by our specialist spinal cord stimulator nurses in an education session that aims to introduce them to the therapy and the technology. This assessment is designed to decide whether the patient would be able to cope with the programming device and with the trial period. Spinal cord stimulation is a relatively straightforward therapy, but a degree of dexterity and technological savvy is required to manage the technology, including the ability to understand and adjust the programmer. The patient's social situation and their ability to care for their surgical wounds is also given consideration and our nurses begin a conversation about rehabilitation and improving function.

Thirdly, patients are assessed by a clinical psychologist. The aim of this appointment is to position the patient's engagement with spinal cord stimulation within the wider context of a philosophy of improving their function and reducing the distress and disability associated with persistent pain. We generally find that patients who are poorly oriented towards improving their quality of life and function do less well with the therapy. We present spinal cord stimulation as a quality-of-life-improving therapy rather than simply a cure for pain; whilst the aim of the therapy is primarily to reduce pain, if the patient does not understand that rehabilitation is the ultimate goal (because we cannot completely obliterate the abnormal sensations) then inserting the device does not achieve the desired outcome. Patients who have high levels of catastrophizing and uncontrolled psychological problems such as psychosis or depression also respond poorly; in my view this is simply because their brain is too overwhelmed to appreciate the change in sensory information reaching it as a result of the spinal cord stimulator's effect.

The psychologist also safety-nets the patients in order to assess how they will cope if the device fails to relieve their pain. Patients often come to us with great expectations (usually because of promises made by a correspondingly distressed surgeon when referring the patient to the pain clinic) and we try to manage and anticipate potential distress should the therapy fail by making the patient aware that the modulation of information from the spinal cord does not necessarily need to occur with the device, but that their ability to manage the situation from a psychological point of view can also influence the sensations they experience. Our psychologists often unearth issues which are not made privy to us clinicians; patients often disclose substance misuse disorders and whether they have contemplated suicide, and the psychologist will sometimes recommend rehabilitation therapies prior to a trial of spinal cord stimulation to give the patient the best chance of having a good outcome. Once all three teams have assessed the patient a decision is made as to whether to proceed with a trial of this device.

Patients are usually referred by our neurosurgical or spinal orthopaedic colleagues who have operated on the patient's spine and, from a technical point of view and based on a repeat MRI scan, have done so successfully, but the patient continues to experience pain. Alternatively, patients are referred by their GPs or by a pain consultant from another service that does not insert the spinal cord stimulation devices, possibly because they do not understand them, although we have made efforts to try to communicate our outcomes to our colleagues. I sometimes think that the individuals and clinics that refer patients for this treatment are reluctant to do so because it is acknowledging that their service is not embracing the wider breadth of pain medicine. In any event our struggle to raise the profile of this therapy, which probably has the best evidence base in all of pain medicine, continues.

Our role as doctors at the point of first contact clinic is to assess whether the individual has the type of pain which would be responsive to spinal cord stimulation, i.e. whether they have neuropathic pain or not. This is not always straightforward; just because you have had a discectomy it does not mean that the pain you had when you presented to the surgeon was due to damage of a nerve. Non-specific lower-back pain with trigger points that form in muscles can mimic the pain from sciatica. Patients consequently go on to have surgery to their spines when they never actually had neuropathic pain. We also assess whether the patient would be medically suitable for a trial of spinal cord stimulation. Uncontrolled diabetes, heavy smoking and reliance on high-dose opioids all pose risks in terms of possible infection and morbidity from the procedure. We assess whether patients would be able to lie flat for the forty-five minutes that it takes to insert the device because, depending on the degree of disability that patients develop due to their pain, this may not be possible. And as mentioned above, we check that the patient is oriented towards improving their quality of life.

Doctors have a duty to inform the patient of their personal experience with a treatment and what their personal complication rates are, so at this initial meeting I will always explain my entry into, experience with and practice in the context of the history of the development of spinal cord stimulation. As doctors we are involved with people at a level where trust is vital and transparency in the face of their adversity is paramount to ensuring satisfactory outcomes. Competence, caring and kindness should be the attitudes which pervade medical care (and life in general).

I was first introduced to spinal cord stimulation in 2007 when I was a trainee at the hospital that I currently work at. I often reflect these days – twenty-two years since graduating from medical school – on how most of my life-changing decisions have come about because of love. I came to the

UK because I ran away from home in order for a relation-ship to survive and I ended up becoming a pain consultant as a result of the pain around the loss of this relationship. It occurred at a time when I was doing my intermediate train-ing in pain medicine and I was at a particularly reflective time in my life, looking to engage long term in understand-ing myself. In 2007 I was in a relationship where I needed to continue to stay in Manchester and I was told that if I wanted a job at the hospital that I am currently at then I would have to learn how to insert and manage spinal cord stimulator devices. So I did.

When I started implanting spinal cord stimulators in 2007, we used systems that relied on producing a pleas-ant tingling sensation (paraesthesia) in the area where the patient usually experienced pain, in order to give some relief; this is known as a paraesthesia-based therapy. The original idea underpinning spinal cord stimulation was that if you were able to produce a tingling sensation in the affected area by placing the electrode over the area of the spinal cord where the nerves that represented that area were situated, then that would result in pain relief. The amount of pain relief was directly proportional to the degree of cov-erage that you got of the painful area. These therapies used low-frequency currents at low amplitudes. You could adjust the pulse width and the amplitude in order to increase the electrical current's depth of penetration into the spinal cord or broaden how many nerve fibres it included. If you imagine a 10-cm wire with a bubble around it, changing the shape of the bubble would allow you to increase the amount of coverage that you had of the patient's painful area. Too big a bubble, however, and you will start to catch the nerves which exit the spinal cord carrying both sensation and movement, which would result in painful muscle contraction. The problem we also had with these paraesthesia-based therapies was that when the patient moved, the spinal cord would float towards or away from the electrode that you had implanted, changing the area, degree and intensity of stimulation that the patient felt because of changes in electrical resistance. The companies involved in manufacturing spinal cord stimulator systems tried to overcome this limitation by producing batteries that could sense the person's position in time and space. When they were upright you could program electrical variables that adjusted for the resistance in that position and you could do the same when they were sitting or standing. This was an attempt to maintain a constant degree of stimulation despite body movement. It worked a bit like your phone whose screen changes from landscape to portrait orientation depending on the way that you hold it. The other challenge, alongside producing constant paraesthesia, was to make sure that the device was compatible with MRI scans, which the patient may need in the future given the increasing usefulness of this technology in detecting, for example, brain haemorrhages, ligament damage and breast cancer.

*

With any new patient the therapy is first trialled before a permanent implant is put in. For reasons that we still don't fully understand, not everybody responds to this therapy. There is some suggestion that the longer you have had your neuropathic pain, the less likely it is that we can influence the damaged nerves. I sometimes explain to patients that their pain is a bit like a bowl of soup: when the bowl of soup is fresh and hot, adding salt and pepper can definitively change the flavour; the longer the soup has stood and become cold and congealed the less likely it is that the addition of salt and pepper will influence the flavour. Unfortunately, we have no way of reheating the soup. The great sadness is that despite the vast evidence base for this therapy and its longevity, patients often come to us after having had their pain for more than four or five years. This statistically holds true across the whole of the UK, and it represents a significant failure to integrate the therapy more effectively into the management of a condition which causes a greater impact on health-related quality of life than cancer, heart or respiratory disease.

I mentioned before that the aim was to try to produce tingling in the affected area in order to provide pain relief. The trial procedure therefore involves placing the lead and subtly changing its position up or down and from side to side over the spinal cord in order to target 100 per cent of the patient's painful area. This could often take a long time in the operating theatre and the difficulty was always that once the patient stood up you could lose stimulation in the area that you had previously obtained tingling in because the lead had moved in relation to the spinal cord or the spinal cord itself, being a mobile structure, had altered its position. The painstaking exercise in theatre of mapping stimulation to the patient's painful area could therefore be lost immediately following their return to the recovery room.

Spinal cord stimulation has evolved as a therapy and the problems above have been laboured at in order to achieve paraesthesia that was predictable and consistent. Better anchors for the leads were made to prevent them from migrating upwards or downwards and therefore losing the area of the spinal cord you wished to stimulate. Batteries were made smaller and rechargeable and MRI-compatible. Programming was made easier with algorithms which were able to more quickly target the nerves that were responsible for sensation to a particular area of the body, and they were also designed so that you could focus the electricity on a particular area such as the foot or the knee. Despite these attempts, over time a percentage of patients would start to dislike the tingling and would start obsessing about the tingling rather than about their pain. The change in tingling with movement was also inhibitory to increasing activity (which was after all a large aspect of the desired outcome) and it was not advised that patients drive with their tingling activated for fear that a sudden uncomfortable burst of stimulation could distract them and cause an accident, nor could patients sleep with the therapy on, which was a major impediment because pain is often worse at night.

From around 2008 rumours began to surface in the spinal cord stimulator community of a new therapy that did not rely on producing tingling to achieve pain relief. Studies were produced that followed up patients who had been implanted with these devices, and they showed results that were hard to believe because they were so good. These were prospective studies in a series of patients, and they were done in centres across Europe by clinicians who are well known for being early adopters of therapies. The idea of spinal cord stimulation using tingling was rooted in the very believable concept of the gate control theory, and the idea that you could have pain relief through a lead implanted in the spinal epidural space that did not rely on tingling was heresy – particularly since the company making the new devices could not provide a clear mechanism of action or explanation for why they should work.

Much work has been done in traditional spinal cord stimulation (as it is now called) in order to elucidate the mechanism of action. This was studied by injuring the sciatic nerves of rats, then implanting little spinal cord stimulators to assess what was happening at the level of the spinal cord. The evidence from these experiments is that wide dynamic range neurones which are made more excitable in neuropathic pain are affected by the activation of the touch fibres. There is also evidence that the stimulation of the spinal cord results in the release of serotonin and noradrenaline which, as we have seen, inhibit the excitable neurones that give rise to pain. Being told that you could achieve pain relief without producing tingling was very much like being told that the Earth revolved around the Sun rather than the Earth being the centre of the universe. The absence of a spaceship to look down on the solar system meant that it was much easier to continue to believe that this was a placebo effect rather than due to a definitive therapeutic benefit.

I have to say that I was on the side of the sceptics when it came to adopting what is now known as high-frequency spinal cord stimulation. This new system, made by a company based in San Jose, uses 10,000 hertz as a frequency. The idea is that this high-frequency current changes the balance of misbehaving nerves in the spinal cord; if we think of the nerves like a class of children, the current empowers those nerves that behave well by increasing their power, which in turn exerts an inhibitory effect on the badly behaved nerves and therefore makes the class of children overall seem better behaved. The tingling-based therapies, on the other hand, make the normal children in the class louder and more distracting, taking attention away from the badly behaved children.

I was approached on a number of occasions by one of the representatives from the company that had produced the 10 kHz paradigm, and we developed a relationship over the years whereby he would continue to bring me the results of the prospective studies and I would continue to doubt, and to express that unless he showed me a mechanism of action or a study that demonstrated superiority of the new therapy over the traditional system then I could not in all good conscience offer it to my patients.

In 2015 the results of a landmark randomized controlled trial were published with a follow-up study of the same cohort of patients published two years later. This study demonstrated that not only was the 10 kHz device not inferior to paraesthesia-based therapies but it was in fact superior in terms of pain relief for back and leg pain in patients with peripheral neuropathic pain due to spine disease. This study represented the largest randomized controlled trial in the history of spinal cord stimulation.

There was much unhappiness and gnashing of teeth at the results of the study, particularly from the companies that had been manufacturing the traditional spinal cord stimulators, and a rapid scrabbling around on their part as they tried to come up with an alternative narrative to what was fundamentally a complete market disruptor. In much the same way that Galileo faced censure when he challenged the prevailing model that had the Earth at the centre of the solar system, the companies producing traditional devices went on full attack. At the centre where I work, my colleague and I sat down quietly and reviewed the scientific paper. We considered the way that the study was conducted and concluded that based on this evidence we had no choice but to offer patients the therapy. We therefore first implanted a patient with a 10 kHz system in 2016. We have to date implanted over a hundred patients and our results have been consistent with the published evidence in terms of pain relief as well as the change in our service delivery. No longer do we spend upwards of an hour and a half mapping tingling in theatre. The procedure now takes about thirty minutes (meaning we are able to implant more patients) and because patients do not have to program the device depending on their position they are able to have it on when they are sleeping or driving, and because it is not affected by the patient's movements it offers no obstruction to the patient embracing their rehabilitation goals.

Paraesthesia-free or paraesthesia-independent spinal cord stimulation, which is what the 10 kHz system represents, now has its competitors. Next to come along was burst stimulation, which purports to have a different mechanism of action whereby it reduces the level at which an individual feels stimulation to just below perception. Newer systems where the lead is placed around the dorsal root ganglion (the exit site of the nerve as it leaves the spinal cord) rather than the spinal cord have been produced in order to focus tingling more effectively. Companies have come up with their own version of paraesthesia-free programming, referring to the total charge delivered rather than the frequency.

The 10 kHz spinal cord stimulator is a great example of a market disruptor. It is no different from the introduction of fruit-named telephones versus those that were produced in Finland. If you produce a therapy overnight that sweeps away the problems associated with the previous therapy, then you can end up with a whole industry in turmoil. People's livelihoods depend on these therapies and their behaviour is dictated accordingly. Relationships have often been established between companies and clinicians who offer a therapy and these relationships sometimes persist in the absence of evidence to support their ongoing use and in the presence of evidence to support the use of a different therapy. NICE has been caught in the midst of this battle, as have various societies that represent pain clinicians, with everyone producing furious arguments and counterarguments. Allegations in whispered tones have even been made about spinal cord injury due to the 10 kHz frequency charge, in order to detract from the delivery of this paradigm-disrupting therapy. In our unit, we quietly continue to collect data following the implantation of 10 kHz devices, not only on pain relief but also on improved sleep, function and reduction in medication use. We inform our patients on potential outcomes based on the information we have collected from patients who have been implanted with this therapy compared to the results of the studies. In our view all we can do is be transparent about our data and continue to monitor the efficacy of the therapy beyond just pain relief.

In our view the ability to engage more actively in reha-bilitation without the distraction of paraesthesia, as well as being able to sleep and drive, are of priceless importance to patients. The 10 kHz therapy also does not require exten-sive programming and we therefore have less cause to bring patients back to clinic which is more convenient for them and for us. Spinal cord stimulation does transform people's lives. It is probably the most satisfying therapy that you can deliver as a pain clinician, and patients literally talk about us having saved their lives. Moreover, it is not an instantaneous therapy; there is a wash-in period where the nerve is being modulated to the point where the patient starts noticing pain relief, which makes us believe that it is not a placebo effect. In addition, the 10 kHz platform can also produce the traditional paraesthesia-based stimulation and a form of burst stimulation. One system to rule them all...

*

I insert spinal cord stimulator trial leads on a Monday morning. It is the best part of my week. I know that there is at least an 85 per cent chance that I will provide the person lying on the operating table with more than 50 per cent pain relief on average. Some patients get close to achieving 100 per cent pain relief.

The implantation takes place at a day-surgery unit. The patient is awake during the procedure, which is done under local anaesthetic. Many patients are uncertain about being awake because of their high levels of anxiety and are concerned about whether they will be able to lie flat. For a long time we used to give patients intravenous sedation and pain relief in order to overcome the inevitable anxiety of having the procedure; now I find that a small oral sedative prior to coming to theatre helps patients with anxiety.

We use an X-ray machine to place the needle in the epidural space. We thread a wire through the epidural needle and, for patients with leg pain, the final lead placement is around the area where a woman's bra strap would be. The exit site where the wire comes out of the skin on the side of the torso is just above the patient's beltline, and the wire is then attached to an external battery. I usually tell patients all sorts of stories whilst they are being operated on; there is often a discussion about politics or the week's events or football or what the patient has done that weekend, designed to distract patients and to enable them to focus on the future. Our spinal cord stimulator nurse sits at the end of the bed and talks to the patient, particularly at times when the procedure may be more uncomfortable. Behind me is the representative from the company who checks that the electrical connections have been made appropriately.

Our spinal cord stimulator team also includes a neuro-surgeon. He provides us with a surgical governance frame-work as non-surgeons. One of the greatest difficulties in the world of neuromodulation is that traditionally implant-ers have been drawn from a subset of needle jockeys within the world of pain medicine and who are trained as anaes-thesiologists. Anaesthesiologists are primarily trained in facilitating surgery by anaesthetizing patients and provid-ing them with pain relief. We usually take a background role and the idea of being at the centre of a therapy is unusual. It often confuses theatre staff when sometimes I'm sat at the anaesthetic machine minding my own busi-ness and at other times I am the one doing the operation. Anaesthesiologists are generally quite risk-averse and we like to live in a world where we control all the elements; for us, failure results in an almost immediate and catastrophic outcome for the patient. Surgeons have a different temperament; they understand the slings and arrows of outrageous fortune that is surgery and can, over time, develop the ability to deal emotionally with complications.

Some units therefore operate a trial system where the pain doctor inserts a temporary lead and, once the trial is completed, the lead is removed. The patient then has to see a neurosurgeon who performs an open and invasive operation under general anaesthetic in order to place a new lead and a permanent battery. Sometimes the patient complains that the outcome following the removal of the trial lead is not the same with the new surgical lead. You therefore have a therapy where the anaesthetic-trained pain doctor is skilled at inserting the percutaneous lead, but the surgeon is not. There are some units where surgeons have learnt how to put in percutaneous leads and do their own trials and insert their own batteries. There are also units, such as ours, which are entirely run by pain doctors who are trained anaesthesiologists, where we insert a permanent lead at trial stage, which then remains in place and is connected to the internal battery that we insert after the trial is complete. There is no standardization in the delivery of neuromodulation.

There has been a great deal of progress made in some countries over the last few years. Some have implemented attempts to standardize education within the field of neuromodulation and established guidance with regards to the minimum acceptable standards of technical competency amongst implanters. They have also tried to actively promote women in neuromodulation, as the number of women working in this area, and in pain medicine generally, does not reflect the more than 50 per cent enrolment of women in medical school and the high number of women in anaesthesiology, where pain medicine draws its trainees from. The uncertainty about the future of pain medicine as a specialty due to the decommissioning of interventional therapies will not, I fear, help this situation and many will opt to just push propofol (an anaesthetic drug) for a living.

Following surgery, patients are then sent back to the day-surgery unit where the device is programmed, and they are given instructions for the next ten days. They keep a diary of their pain scores and how they feel during the trial. I see the patient again on the following Wednesday, but our nurses ring them on the Friday, by which time we usually know whether the trial has been successful or not. Spinal cord stimulation with paraesthesia-based therapies is a bit like Marmite – patients either love it or hate it – but with 10 kHz there is just a resigned disappointment if the therapy fails to deliver 50 per cent pain relief. Those patients who experience pain relief find the therapy transformative. Their partners will often say they have been less grumpy, and the patients sometimes say that for the first time they have been able to feel their feet again and that they were able to walk without a stick. It really is the most gratifying therapy that you can be involved with.

If the patient has achieved more than 50 per cent pain relief then ten days after the insertion of the trial, we cut the external wire. Patients are often quite distressed because they know that in around forty-eight hours' time their pain will have returned. We then insert the permanent battery the following Monday. The theatre procedure is the same, only this time a small pocket is made in the patient's back just above the buttocks for the battery. The battery measures approximately 4 x 3 cm and is about 1 cm thick. It is inserted under the skin and, depending on how fat the patient is, may or may not be visible. Patients then take about two weeks to heal and after that they have a permanent device (and a special card to present at airport security).

We see the patients two weeks later to check that their wounds are okay and then we see them at three, six and twelve months. We therefore witness a gradual transformation in somebody who was not able to do very much, was depressed and potentially going to lose their jobs. One of my patients used to be a rugby coach and when I first saw him he had lost this role and the social life that came with it. He felt unable to participate in day-to-day activities and was struggling at his workplace. Initially he was quite unsure about whether a spinal cord stimulator was for him. He went to see a pain management physiotherapist who reassured him that his spine was structurally safe and started to get him to exercise gradually but he continued to struggle with the neuropathic pain in his leg. Eventually he decided to go forward and have the spinal cord stimulator trial. He had a very successful trial and when I saw him the other day in the waiting room, he hurried up to me and said that he was refereeing rugby again. He has regained his sense of humour and is back to doing what he loves. A little bit of electricity has facilitated this change.

Another of my patients is a policeman. He sustained an injury at work and was unable to walk because of constant pain. His mobility was improved by surgery, but his leg pain continued. He struggled for years taking medication which did not help with his pain but affected his ability to think and concentrate. He said that he really struggled to drive, and he also picked up weight because of his inability to do any exercise. He was having spinal injections every six months and he says they took a fraction of the pain away, but they were never completely effective. He had a trial of spinal cord stimulation and he has now lost three stone in weight. He says that apart from the very small scars on his back you wouldn't even know that he had a device. He says that he has now obtained over 90 per cent pain relief and must charge the device for around thirty minutes every day. He says he also hasn't had any time off work since having the device put in.

*

In 2015 I was invited to the headquarters of the company whose paraesthesia-based systems we had been using for many years. The aim of the visit was to meet with their scientists to discuss the therapy and to tour the factory where the equipment was manufactured. I found the factory tour illuminating because I had grown up with a penchant for watching TV programmes about how things were made. The tour gave me a better understanding of the challenges involved in manufacturing the equipment and the rigorous safety standards involved. I also met the inventors of what I think is the world's greatest spinal cord stimulator lead anchoring system and visited the 3D-printing lab where they had devised the equipment. Despite no longer using the rest of the company's equipment I continue to use the anchor.

As part of the visit to the factory I was also taken to the annual meeting of the North American Neuromodulation Society (NANS). This meeting is held annually in Las Vegas, which I am told is because even the smallest city in the US has a direct flight to Sin City. I had never been to an American medical meeting. They are so much more fun than any European or British meeting and massive in scale. I sat in the audience of the opening ceremony – and I call it an opening ceremony deliberately because it was like the Olympics – when the lights suddenly dimmed and there was the blaring of triumphant rock music. The organizers of the meeting all stepped out on to the stage with their profile pictures and qualifications revolving on the cinematic projection screen behind them. It was unlike any conferences or meetings held in the UK.

The reason why the NANS conference is good is because the American market for spinal cord stimulation makes up

50 per cent of the world's total spinal cord stimulator revenue, with the remainder of the first world making up the rest, and therefore anything that is new or interesting is likely to be presented at the US meeting. It was at this conference that our pain clinic started its journey with paraesthesia-independent spinal cord stimulation because it was where the author of the study presented the preliminary results of the randomized control trial on high-frequency spinal cord stimulation versus paraesthesia-based stimulation. Based on my assessment of the presentation I decided that I should probably give more consideration to his therapy. The scientific paper of that presentation was then published later that year. Interestingly, at that meeting were a group of people promoting a new spinal cord stimulator therapy, but they could only talk to European and British doctors because the rules laid down by the Food and Drug Administration in America meant that no American doctor could speak to them yet as the therapy had not been approved. They were therefore there in full view of anyone passing by but could not engage with any American doctors, and there were even monitors there to check that they didn't talk to one another. Weird.

Now that we have entered the age of paraesthesia-free therapies there has been a mammoth gunfight in terms of coming up with competition to the 10 kHz system. There have even been court battles with regards to whether you can patent a frequency. Papers have been written which have sought to undermine 10 kHz as an effective therapy.

Trials have been hastily put together to indicate that 10 kHz is no better than 1 kHz and that the therapy consists largely of a placebo response. Mud has been slung and evidence interrogated. I spoke at a meeting the other day and at the end of my talk one of the attendees said to me, in an open forum, 'I'm very happy for you, but remember these guys' – the company whose therapy I was talking about – 'are bastards. There's a reason why their share price is dropping, and you will find that their batteries don't last very long.' This criticism came from a very experienced implanter. My response to him was that based on our implementation of the therapy and unceasing collecting of data, as well as the published evidence, all I could do is hope that the company is acting in good faith in terms of the therapy. He came up to me privately after the meeting to apologize for his remarks and wished me well. I was interested to note that his main preoccupation appeared to be with the share price of the company, and I was later told that he had invested quite heavily in the company and had lost money accordingly with the vagaries of the stock exchange.

There is a lot of money to be made in terms of implanting devices – in persistent pain and generally in medicine. Chronic pain is a global problem and, as I mentioned earlier in the chapter, neuropathic pain affects 6 to 8 per cent of people within any given population. For a long time paraesthesia-based therapies dominated the spinal cord stimulator market and the competition between companies was all around how slick their programming was in theatre and after the implant was inserted permanently, so that patients could be optimized in terms of getting the tingling in the right place. There was huge competition between manufacturers in terms of the battery size, how quickly it would charge and how long it would last – some manufacturers had batteries with definite failure dates meaning that they could guarantee that a replacement would need to be bought. At the mercy of all these shenanigans is the patient. Companies fight amongst themselves to the detriment of therapies that have a good evidence base and clinicians fight amongst themselves to the detriment of patients. Government organizations which rely on clinicians to provide them with objective opinions are therefore confounded.

The last ten years have been a constant struggle for me in the world of neuromodulation. I have had to struggle to reform the unit that I work in with regards to implementing a robust quality assurance framework in terms of infection control policies and operational policies whilst continuing to develop my own skills. I have had to get all our psychologists on board and try to situate the therapy within the context of a disability and stress reduction model and I have had to train another colleague in inserting these devices. I have had very little help from the world of neuromodulation, and in many ways my experience has been that those who are the most experienced in implanting are more concerned with jumping on the next research bandwagon, in order to improve their profiles and line their pockets or inflate their egos, than they have been in ensuring that patients have greater access to the therapy and that the next generation of implanters are trained and appropriately supported. I have heard stories about clinicians in senior education positions within pain medicine who continue to use paraesthesia-based therapies because they feel that the skill of an implanter is in their ability to place the lead, ensuring that paraesthesia is produced that covers the patient's entire pain area – not in placing a lead over a defined vertebral level. This attitude is held and expounded in the presence of high-quality evidence that demonstrates that paraesthesia-free therapies are superior.

The evidence is the evidence – not at all perfect but in the words of the philosopher Karl Popper (1902–1994), 'our aim as scientists is objective truth; more truth, more interesting truth, more intelligible truth. We cannot reasonably aim at certainty ... Since we can never know anything for sure, it is simply not worth searching for certainty; but it is well worth searching for truth; and we do this chiefly by searching for mistakes, so that we can correct them.'

I think it is churlish and disingenuous to demand rigorous scientific studies, which a randomized control trial aims to be, in order to prove objectively that one therapy is superior to another or has an effect over and above a placebo response and then to turn around and say that actually the 'in my hands' argument has greater weight. The expression 'in my hands' is often used by doctors who believe that, despite the results of scientific studies that have tried to reduce bias, their personal experience of implanting thirty to fifty patients and collecting (oftentimes retrospective) data supersedes the controlled trial with its attempts to minimize bias.

We still use paraesthesia-based stimulation in our unit, alongside the newer treatment, because we believe that stimulation therapies are iterative, and so we offer patients the option of whichever device we believe they should trial based on an assessment of their clinical problem. What is important to patients includes not only pain relief but also the impact on their daily life, such as whether they will be able to drive with a therapy or sleep with it on.

*

In a time when interventional pain therapies are becoming more and more rationed in terms of their provision because the evidence base is so poor for them, neuromodulation in the form of spinal cord stimulation is probably the best evidence-based interventional therapy, but it is not always available for patients. Pain medicine is in crisis as a specialty. Due to the rationing of radiofrequency procedures and facet joint injections as well as the closing of units that provide only interventional services, we are losing people and not attracting a new generation to the specialty. Neurosurgeons are generally not interested in functional neurosurgery in the form of implanting spinal cord stimulators and the lack of pain doctors becoming implanters means that a therapy which has a robust evidence base and life-changing outcome is not being supported.

A therapy that is not life-saving but aims to improve quality of life is easily sidelined if it is not championed. This is less of an issue in a society where healthcare is provided privately, and is driven by the incentive for doctors to provide therapies in order to earn themselves a living, but in a publicly funded healthcare system where we depend on the government to decide which therapies are offered and where we are not taking responsibility for the consistent and national delivery of evidence-based therapies, we are very vulnerable. The challenge in private healthcare systems, on the other hand, is to curtail the enthusiasm of doctors when it comes to trialling patients. The trial to successful implantation ratio in some of these privately funded systems, for example, is around 40 per cent, whereas in the UK's public sector it tends to run between 70 and 90 per cent. It is not hard to see that in a private system where you get paid for every patient you trial there may be a financial incentive to trial patients who might not be suitable.

We have colleagues who continue to think of spinal cord stimulation as voodoo. Despite greater evidence than we have for any of the rehabilitation therapies that we offer, this belief that the Earth is flat and that the Sun revolves around the Earth continues to be perpetuated by clinicians who, for various reasons, refuse to accept the difference that this form of pain relief can make to a patient's life. The traditional view from a behaviourist point of view is that in chronic pain management the aim is not to reduce pain but to improve function. This mantra unfortunately leads some clinicians to abandon the pursuit of pain relief. Ultimately, however, it is merely two sides of the same coin, because both spinal cord stimulation and rehabilitation therapies aim to modulate the nervous system. Whether neuromodulation is brought about by drugs, electricity or talking, the outcome for the patient is the same: an improvement in quality of life and an improvement in the ability of an individual to serve their communities and their families. Socrates is credited with having said, 'The only thing I know is that I know nothing' – as I get older this is the only certainty I believe in the practice of medicine, and in life generally.

Do not go gentle into that good night

Getting older is of course inevitable, and for some the aches and pains which are experienced, and the changes in their body, are simply perceived as a normal part of ageing. Gradually people contract their world, it becomes smaller and smaller as their ability to function diminishes. My father and I were having a discussion along these lines this morning. I asked him how he was feeling, and he said that he was feeling 'subpar'. My dad is seventy-three, although he rounds his age up to seventy-five when he thinks we are not taking him seriously. He has acquired the diseases of a well-lived life and is on the associated medications that accompany these maladies. He is restricted in terms of taking some medications because they can interact with his prescribed drugs and he must avoid certain foods which can elevate his blood sugar or precipitate an attack of gout. He does push the envelope when it comes to his gout and diabetes, and sometimes the temptation of meat or an ice-cream float is too much.

He said that in his surgery that morning he had seen a few 73-year-olds who were slipping gradually into dementia. He was reflecting on why some people in their seventies appear to be able to soldier on whilst others – and here he used an Afrikaans word – are *inmekaar*, which literally translates as 'folded in on themselves'. I mused that in my experience individuals who continue to engage in work, keeping their brains from atrophying, and who remain socially engaged are less likely to experience this gradual decline. I also said to him that people who continue to exercise and use their muscles are less likely to experience physical atrophy. I have noticed that some people give up on living as they get older, and I think that this programs their cells to start committing ritual suicide. I told my father that the reason he has not declined into dementia and is not *inmekaar* is probably because he has continued to work as a GP. (I later went into the house and my mum told me that the reason he was feeling subpar was in fact because his gout was playing up.)

The elderly patients I see in the UK tend to fall into one of two groups: a group that is aggressively pursuing health by regularly going to the gym and spending a large part of the day doing mental puzzles, and a contrasting group that appears to be waiting at St Peter's gate on a permanent basis. These two groups seek healthcare for very different purposes: the former group is looking for a functional improvement and the latter group is looking for palliation and comfort. For those who choose to *not* go gentle into that good night this gradual decline associated with abnormal feedback from their bodies is unacceptable and they sally forth seeking a cure. Intolerance with inevitable ageing has resulted in an explosion of the medicalization of ageing and aggressive marketing of wellness (in South Africa there is a chain of health shops called the Wellness Warehouse). There is an adage that reads: We ruin our health in search of wealth, to seek, to have, to save, and then we spend our wealth in search of health only to find the grave.

Older adults like my father live on the edge when it comes to health and well-being. Failure of organ systems, including heart failure and kidney disease, as well as diseases like chronic obstructive pulmonary disease, may result in the experience of chronic pain, and drugs used to alleviate this pain may not work as well or their use may result in unanticipated side effects which make the consequences of treating the condition harder to bear than the condition itself. The older person's nervous system changes, and this has implications with regards to the experience of pain. The fatty layer of the nerves in the spinal cord is reduced and there are fewer connections within the brain, particularly in those areas involved in the processing of information about tissue damage. Age also brings with it a decrease in the body's naturally occurring opioids which help regulate pain without any intervention. Despite these changes, however, it is unclear whether these physiological alterations cause a difference in the pain response of the older person to harmful stimuli. They may offer some evidence of very minor increases in the ability of the older person to resist mild pain as they get older, or this evidence may merely reflect greater stoicism by the older adult (or fear of an 'I told you so' from their children when gout visits) and their belief that pain and discomfort are an inevitable consequence of advancing years.

What we do know is that older patients report less pain, or pain in a different distribution, compared to young adults with the same clinical problem. Pain assessment may be difficult in the older person because of changes in cognition along with reduced memory and an inability or incapacity to report pain due to dementia; we have therefore developed specific pain scales which rely on factors other than self-report to assess the experience of pain. Restlessness, grimacing or sounds such as grunting or groaning may point to an individual being in pain. These non-specific behaviours are difficult to make sense of, however, and managing pain in the context of an individual who is unable to report what they are feeling is challenging. The struggle is to avoid responding by giving patients aggressive quantities of usually opiate-based analgesics, rendering them more vulnerable to the complications of these medications, versus grappling with the fear that we are leaving somebody to suffer.

Chronic pain has a significant effect on patients who are older. It results in reduced mobility and avoidance of activities and may cause individuals to fall due to their inability to rapidly change position as a result of pain. The consequent impact on the individual's ability to function may lead to depression and anxiety. Family and social relationships are disrupted and chronic pain in older adults places a significant burden on the communities within which these individuals live. Increasing social isolation and a reduced capacity for travel impacts on the ability of older adults to access services, and stoicism and not wanting to bother the doctor also play a role. One of the most pressing challenges in the management of older adults with chronic pain is access to rehabilitation therapies in the form of behavioural interventions and physical reactivation and conditioning.

*

Spouses have always played a significant role in the management of patients with persistent pain. Their role is fundamental in the delivery of emotional support because they are the patient's constant companion, as the following story of Alan and Louise illustrates. With patients in their later years many have lost their lifelong spouse or partner, or their partner may not be able to support them practically.

Dear Abdul

Well I think after twelve years I can call you that – under the circumstances. I just want to thank you for all that you've done for Louise over the twelve years. As for no doubt she would have been in a wheelchair if it wasn't for you. I hope now that you are Professor Lalkhen – I hope that you won't stop seeing Louise as you know she will not let anyone else do her treatment. Well Professor I'm sorry I will not be seeing you again. I hope you will carry on doing the good work that you do and have a good life. Carry on taking care of your mum and dad like our Michael will do with Louise. I enclose a small gift to you which I hope you accept. With kind regards for all that you have done.

Best wishes,
Alan

Alan and Louise always came to see me for her clinic review appointment together and have done so since they both retired. They would drive all the way from North Wales, which is outside our catchment area but I continued to see and treat Louise after they moved there, having first met them whilst I was still a trainee doctor and they were living in England, much closer to my pain clinic. When I became a consultant, I continued to see Louise and perform her then four-monthly steroid lumbar and local anaesthetic injections into her spine joints. Louise is my patient, but over the years Alan became my friend.

I received this letter from Alan, delivered by Louise on the day of her next scheduled injection. Louise had rung a few months earlier to let us know that Alan had been diagnosed with lung cancer and had been told that he had not long to live. Louise spoke to my secretary who has been with me since I started as a consultant (in fact I insisted – as much as one can in a publicly funded organization – that having Julie as my secretary was a condition of my employment). Over the years Julie has grown close to Louise, even though they have never met, because Julie arranges the dates for the patient's next injection, and both of us have always received Christmas gifts from Louise.

Twelve years is a long time to know anyone, and patients become part of the texture and colour of your life as a doctor and as a person without you even realizing it. Usually injections are performed every four to six months and review appointments are arranged perhaps once or twice a year. Each interaction represents a snapshot in the life of the person you are treating, and in the same way that comparing photographs taken months apart allows you to appreciate change more accurately, this pattern of interaction facilitates a clearer view of the inexorable progression of time and its impact on form and feeling than is often the case with people you see on a day-to-day basis. The snapshots tend to make more of an impression and the changes appear more dramatic. I see my parents who live in South Africa three or four times a year and my anxiety about this infrequent interaction makes me more aware of the changes that they are going through in the same way that I am mindful of how my patients are changing – not just in terms of the pain conditions they present with but in the context of their overall ageing process and the inevitable decline that is associated with this.

One of the reasons I think that I decided to embrace pain medicine as a subspecialty of anaesthesia was perhaps because of this yearning for a relationship longer than the five minutes it takes to ask about gastroesophageal reflux, last meal eaten and previous anaesthetic history, which is usually the sum of an anaesthesiologist's conversation with a patient before surgery. I think sometimes as doctors we feel that these interactions do not touch us and that patients pass through our hands without leaving an impression, but I remember unfolding the piece of paper with Alan's hand-written note and reading the words and realizing how much he had come to mean to me. Even though it was Louise who was my patient, I always took the opportunity when seeing them to gently admonish Alan about his smoking. During the time I knew him he had treatment for coronary artery disease and he suffered with numerous chest infections, but never missed attending an appointment with his wife. Our common ground was a discussion around cars and Alan found it amusing that I moved from owning various cars to eventually giving up cars altogether and riding a bicycle. His final parting gift to me was a watch and a bicycle pump. I remember sitting down in my office and reading his note and I could almost hear his laboured breathing and see his ready smile as he wrote it. I found myself unexpectedly crying as I sat at my desk.

I saw Louise some months later for her regular spine injection. Louise is extremely thin and has struggled with osteoporotic fractures of her back, which means that over time the bones of her spine have thinned out and as a result they have collapsed under their own weight, changing the shape of her spine and resulting in an abnormal and painful curve in her upper back. These areas become painful because of inflammation between the joints of the spine. She had struggled with lower-back pain for several years, which I treated with steroid and local anaesthetic injections. Over time the pain would flit from her lower back to her neck and then to the mid-section of her back where her fractures were. She would come and see me in between injections and I would prescribe appropriate medication where it helped her, as well as general advice relating to movement, particularly with regards to activity pacing, which she always found challenging. Alan and I would talk about cars, his comments being either derisive or complimentary, depending on the type of car I was then driving. Louise would also complain about Alan and his failure to heed advice with regards to his own health and I would have to referee between the two of them, trying my best not to get involved with either when it came to this issue. I learnt about love and tolerance and respect from Alan and Louise. They were like a well-rehearsed duo, finishing each other's sentences and seamlessly picking up each other's thoughts, producing a stream of loving consciousness. I would often say very little during the consultations, preferring to listen.

At the time of her injection following Alan's death Louise was wearing a formal black dress. She was still extremely upset, and I had asked the day-surgery nurses to make sure she was placed in a side room whilst she waited. I remember sitting with her for a long time, reminiscing about Alan and his passing. She seemed even more gaunt than usual, sunken into herself, and appeared to be struggling to find the energy to carry on without him. It was almost as if by wearing the black dress she was clinging to the memory of her last contact with him, which would have been his funeral. She had decided not to leave Wales and move in with her son who lives closer to the hospital that I work at, because at least in the village in Wales she has friends, whereas if she moved back to England, she would be alone all day. Her son now comes to appointments with her, taking the place of Alan. I last saw her just before Christmas and she admitted that she was coping poorly without Alan and that this time of the year was pregnant with memories that threatened to overwhelm her. The pain of loss and loneliness may well be harder to bear than the pain from an ageing body.

Bereavement and loss are ever-present companions in life but more so with advancing age. I have now been a consultant for a decade and many of my patients when I first started were already in their late sixties and seventies. They are now losing husbands and wives and sometimes children. Sometimes when Julie phones up to arrange their next injection, we are told that the patient themselves has passed away. The passing of the patient's loved ones impacts on their pain experience by changing their ability to suppress the abnormal sensations coming from their bodies and curbing their desire and motivation to carry on regardless. Their losses also impact on me. Sometimes it feels as if I am walking with a group of people whose numbers are ever diminishing. I tell Alan's story because I know he would have wanted me to communicate how challenging it is to support someone who suffers with persistent pain but also to leave a legacy of his great love for Louise. She wants me to tell his story because of her great love for him. It is these stories that make working in this field a privilege.

*

Grace is ninety-four and she always wears a suit when she comes to clinic appointments. She is nearly doubled over but refuses to use a walking aid because she says that it makes her feel old. When she comes to clinic, she is always apologetic because she says that my time could be better spent looking after older patients. Over time Grace's spine has remodelled, as spines generally tend to do. I explain to patients that when they are young (and I mean twenty years old or less) their spines are like cars in a showroom. Over time and with use the car's paintwork fades and the car bears the scars of its interaction with the environment. Whilst the car and the spine continue to function, they no longer look like that showroom version. Studies have shown that age-related changes occur in the spine from your twenties, and these changes are described with words that inspire fear such as disc protrusion, disc bulges, degeneration, nerve compression and facet joint degeneration. As previously touched upon, however, these changes are also apparent in patients who have no pain from their spine area, leading doctors to conclude that none of us retain a showroom spine as we grow older and, frustratingly, that it is difficult to relate back pain to changes found on an MRI scan.

Grace's spine looks like a classic car that has not been lovingly cared for. She has age-related changes in the architecture of her neck and the bones have remodelled and altered to the point where they are compressing on the collection of nerves called the cauda equina (or 'horse's tail') that extends from the bottom part of the spinal cord. Surgery to correct the deformity in her lower back would be a massive undertaking and because of all her complex medical problems she would probably not leave the hospital following such a procedure. Her main complaint is that her legs feel numb and she doesn't always know where they are in space and time. She says that she develops pain in them as she walks, and this limits her ability to shop and do her chores. She also cannot stand when she bakes, and she keenly feels this loss of an activity which made her the centre of a social circle. She has tried many of the medications that we normally use for nerve pain, but they have either made her too sleepy or muddled or constipated.

Grace attends the clinic with her son and daughter, who are both in their late sixties. Her son has had knee replacements and walks with a cane. I find it poignant that her children are so old, but I suppose when you are ninety-four your children can easily be in their seventies. Her children are around the same age as my parents and part of me hopes that I will be able to attend a clinic with my parents in the way that Grace's son and daughter do. She retains much of the fierceness that I suspect made her formidable in her youth. Looking back at the challenges she has faced in her life it emerges that she struggled significantly with mental health problems in her thirties and forties. I think that there is a tendency, and I often reproach the trainees for falling into this trap, to refer to 94-year-old women as cute, as if their advancing age somehow returns them to a second childhood. It is quite easy to forget that the same challenges which patients experienced when they were younger in terms of maladaptive patterns of behaviour follow them into old age. Anxiety and depression, which exacerbate the experience of pain, have the same effect when individuals are older as when they are younger. Unfortunately, what does change with age is the cognitive flexibility to solve problems, as well as the ability to access therapies that are more readily available to younger patients suffering with psychological disorders.

The consultation and conversation I have with Grace and her children mainly involves explaining why she has the weakness in her legs as well as the shooting pain. I explain that these pains are not dangerous and that the best thing to do is to try to maximize the level of activity she is able to do and to understand that the more frustrated and discouraged she becomes the worse her pain will be. She finds some comfort in an explanation which allows her to manage her anxiety at what is becoming an ever-shrinking world. She says to me that she feels as if she is looking through a window and what she can see is becoming more and more faint. The explanation I give her will have to suffice in the absence of being able to offer her definitive treatment for her nerve pain and leg weakness. We talk to her as a group – me, her daughter and her son – about how helpful we think walking with a frame would be, but she simply tuts at us. Her son's eyes spark with frustration and resignation at a look that he has probably received from his mother all his life, which fortunately for him has been well into his late sixties.

It is not always the case that we cannot offer older patients any form of interventional treatment. Grace's management contrasts with that of Maria, who is eighty-four and looks disconcertingly youthful, so that I sometimes have to remind myself of her age. She is a small woman, always smartly dressed and has a beautifully cut black bob hairstyle. She always wears a full face of make-up. Maria has nerve pain in her right leg because the outlet of one of the nerves in the bottom of her spine has become gradually narrowed. I treat her nerve compression with a steroid injection around this nerve every six months, which allows her to continue to live independently. She lives alone and does all her own housework, including arranging the ends of the Persian carpets on her floors so that they all line up. She travels across the country frequently and has an active social circle. The six-monthly injections to 'discipline' her 'badly behaved' nerve, as she calls it, are her lifeline she says. The point of these stories is that effective pain management must be tailored to the individual and be flexible around them. It also highlights that small interventions have the ability to translate into significant gains in independence.

*

The average age of patients that I list for repeat injection of local anaesthetic and steroid injections for lower-back pain is seventy-seven. Whilst there may be no relationship between the way that a patient's spine looks on an MRI scan and the presence of back pain, nerve pain radiating down an arm or a leg is a different matter and there may be a correlation between what is seen on a scan and the sufferer's pain, which usually occurs within the normal anatomical distribution of that nerve. Spines remodel over the years and new bone is laid down in places where bone should not be created; nerve canals that were once capacious become narrow and impinge on nerves. The problem, however, is not always mechanical, and surgery to relieve the pressure around the nerves does not always result in a pain-free patient. In these cases it may be that the nerve has already been damaged by the pressure exerted on it, like a peach which is compressed; whilst the skin of the peach may look unbroken the flesh below has been bruised and damaged. I often explain to patients that whilst nerves are like cables from the outside, internally they are made up of millions of fragile tubes which are easily disrupted. This narrowing, which is called spinal stenosis, occurs in the lumbar region and compression of the nerves within this canal acts as if you are turning off the flow of water in a dam and so less water is reaching the periphery. The compression is dynamic, and patients will describe being able to walk a certain distance before the narrowing becomes so severe that the flow of water, as it were, ceases altogether, causing them to feel weakness but more often pain in their legs. They then must rest a while to allow the swelling to reduce, the water to begin to flow again, and then they can carry on walking. This is called their claudication distance. Patients describe how they can no longer perform activities at their previous pace and are slowed down. The more active somebody was in their life the more intolerant they tend to be of this kind of limiting pain and consequent loss of function. Injection of a steroid into the nerve canal sometimes relieves the pain, but the evidence for this therapy is poor and it is now no longer recommended by NICE in the UK. There are patients, however, who are intolerant of medication and are unsuitable for surgery where this injection is the only therapy which will help them to function.

One such patient suffering from this narrowing of the spinal canal is ninety years old, only about four feet tall and has come to the clinic today with her daughter, who is seventy, and her grandson, who is probably nearly forty. She has a reduction in the diameter of the spinal column containing the spinal cord in her neck and the cord is being strangled like a river choked by overgrown vegetation along its banks. She constantly feels like she is holding grit in her hands because the nerve signals are not properly getting through to where they should be. She says she sometimes talks to her hands and tells them 'don't be so soft', whilst she tries to wipe this non-existent grit away. Unfortunately she would not be able to tolerate a major operation on her neck and so has to live with this feeling of grittiness in her hands and an inability to hold anything properly. Her walking is also affected but she says that she is too young for a Zimmer frame. She is frustrated because she still lives alone and wants to do her own gardening – her mind and her body have failed to keep pace with one another. The family is quite protective and worries about her because she has been with them for so long that they cannot possibly imagine a time when she would not be part of their lives.

She has tried lots of medications to manage her symptoms, all of which have made her hallucinate, and today we agree that she should take a low dose of codeine combined with paracetamol. She is initially quite reluctant when I say she can take up to eight tablets a day. After I have warned her of the possibility of constipation with this medication, she tells me that eating chocolate now gives her diarrhoea. I respond by saying that if I ever reach ninety and can no longer eat chocolate because it gives me diarrhoea then they can take me away. She laughs at this. I tell her to take the codeine regularly with three bars of chocolate.

Despite her pain and discomfort, together with her growing inability to self-care and be independent, she laughs. It always amazes me at how indomitable the human spirit can be in the face of adversity.

*

We don't really understand why human beings suffer with pain in the joints as they get older. Non-specific lower-back pain is sometimes attributed to the changes that occur in the small joints between individual vertebrae as a person ages, a condition referred to as facet joint pain or facet joint arthropathy. The cartilage within joints does not have a nerve supply and therefore feels no sensation, and the belief is that the abnormal deformation of the joints is what results in the pain because the brain perceives the joint to be in danger; this probably accounts for why weight loss helps with chronic knee-joint pain, and the same may well be true of the lower back. The changes seen on X-rays and MRI scans of the facet joints and the knees have led to therapies that focus on these areas. The knee is a relatively simple target and replacement joints have been created, but this is less practical in the spine, and the equivalent treatment was once considered to be fusion surgery of the lumbar spine or replacement of the intervertebral disc. Both these procedures, however, have been shown to not improve chronic lower-back pain and have since been abandoned. The facet joints are most active when you lean backwards, which has been used as a sign that the lower-back pain experienced by the individual is due to a pathological

issue at the facet joint. Bending, sitting, standing and twisting all become associated with pain. The change is gradual
over many years and the impact is felt with activities that
are innocuous to anyone who does not have pain – changing the duvet cover can become a major hurdle in life. All
of my patients are fiercely independent and despite the
passage of time and the loss of loved ones they prefer to
continue living by themselves rather than moving in with
a relative. Often, they are accompanied by caring and desperate children who want their parents to come and live
with them, only to be met with the refusal to be a burden
or a desire to continue to have their own space. The injection of local anaesthetic and steroids into the facet joints of
elderly patients is thus an important therapy, but because
of the poor evidence base associated with this therapy it is
becoming increasingly difficult to fund it.

There is no explanation for why patients report benefit
from an injection of local anaesthetic and steroid into a
joint where we understand the pain to in fact be due to
changes with the function of the nervous system; an injection into the facet joint should therefore not make any difference to the individual's pain. But for some patients it
does, and it provides a means of coping with pain, although
some say that it does not reduce the pain completely and
over a period of six months the effect gradually wanes.
There are individuals within the scientific community
who attest to the effect being due to placebo and the activation of descending inhibitory pathways triggered by the

patient's belief in the therapy. Some argue that the effect of the steroid has a knock-on impact on the desensitization of the nervous system. I sometimes wonder if all they really benefit from is the continuity of care, knowing that a doctor will see them on a regular basis who will provide a safety net for what they perceive to be their inevitable and inexorable decline into needing to be looked after.

We are now restricted in terms of who we can offer facet joint injections to. Failure of the medical community to establish exactly which patients benefit from this therapy has potentially resulted in the loss of a useful tool. Unfortunately, this procedure has been used inappropriately in young patients where the aim of pain management should instead be to rehabilitate the individual utilizing an approach that recognizes the distress and disability caused by chronic pain and attempts to reverse this situation through a process of cognitive behavioural therapy combined with exercise. Unfortunately, we have also failed older adults in combining these therapies with reactivation of muscles through the provision of activities designed to maintain and improve muscle function and joint flexibility, as this may not be suitable for those in their later years. For some patients, as they get older these injections literally save their lives.

A little club sometimes forms because the patients tend to come for their injections at the same time. I will often wander into the day-care unit where patients are admitted for these procedures to find that the patient is not at his or her bed. I find the patients chatting in groups of three or four with some of their injection clubmates. Little social circles are formed, and friendships are made around their shared treatment and suffering. I am often asked where so-and-so is if they are not at their usual injection slot and sometimes, sadly, I must inform the friend that their fellow injection attendee is no longer with us. The news is greeted with a resigned and sad inevitability and the unspoken knowledge that one day they themselves may well be spoken of in the same way.

Most of my patients tend to be women simply because they live longer than men. I often spend a lot of time comforting patients whose husbands have died. There is no way to capture the depth of loss associated with a friendship which has lasted for more than five decades. When you speak to somebody who has lost a life partner of this duration it is as if too much water has been added to a watercolour; the person becomes indistinct and blurred, with none of the vibrancy that they once had. They are still there in front of you, but the difference is palpable. The adjustment to no longer being in a partnership is difficult to say the least and is often associated with a significant exacerbation of their usual pain symptoms. After her husband died one of my patients got herself a dog and was convinced that the dog was the living reincarnation of her husband in that many of the dog's mannerisms mimicked those of her husband. I often ask patients who have been together for a long time about marriage. I think that in older people we have a repository of knowledge which we often fail to access. I also find the older patients more reflective about their pain and more understanding of the limitations of the science of suffering.

I make no secret of the fact that the assessment and management of the older patients is the part of my job that I enjoy the most. Providing pain management interventions in the form of injections, and sometimes more advanced therapies such as spinal cord stimulation, to the older adult is rewarding and met with a simple gratitude which I find unceasingly humbling. Older patients are like ancient trees that have witnessed the passage of time, and like trees that have borne fruit, the branches are often lower. The lowering of the branches is due to an understanding of the fact that possessions and achievements pass and that what you are left with is the character you have built over time. This is usually not the case in younger patients who are struggling with the burdens of child-rearing and engaging in productive economic activity and where chronic pain is either a vehicle to a living or an impediment to success.

A list of patients in their seventies and eighties for injections is a pleasure; I am always met with a courtesy and respect that I do not often enjoy in other aspects of my professional life. Patients are grateful for any small measure of improvement that they receive in terms of therapy. The older patient tends to still dress up for their clinic appointment and I often remark upon what they wear. I suppose not being in a workplace means that they have wardrobes full of clothes that were once used for a work life and which are now no longer worn. Older patients also tend not to answer their mobile phones during clinic appointments and often have stories to tell and offer a perspective on life which facilitates learning. There is less of a sense of entitlement and more of a sense of gratitude. During the appointment I often see flashes of the personality that once was, and I think that working with older adults in the context of a pain clinic has allowed me to realize that true value comes from how you treat other people and what you are able to give to others. My older patients take an active interest in the changes in my own life situation and curiously always ask after my parents – probably because I frequently talk about them. My parents are often going through some of the same changes that my patients are experiencing and a bridge is formed between caring for the person in my clinic and looking back home.

Pain in older adults is a difficult and challenging societal problem. Chronic pain in the elderly results in an inability to function on a day-to-day basis. The signs of neglect are often there when one examines patients who are living by themselves. Meals are smaller and less complex and weight loss is often a significant issue. Loss of muscle results in an even greater reduction in the capacity to perform activities that require power. The world of the older person becomes smaller as their ability to walk is limited by pain. Holidays which were once looked forward to are no longer possible because health conditions make obtaining insurance difficult. What is often sad is that persistent pain in the older adult is viewed by both providers and by the patients themselves as an untreatable inevitability. Patients therefore must cope with pain and the unavoidable loss of spouses and function as well as a society that ignores and marginalizes them whilst it values the shiny and new.

There is also the problem that, as previously discussed, medication for the management of pain is poorly tolerated with advancing age; there is a change in the sensitivity of receptors, and interaction with drugs used for other diseases of the older adult are common and sometimes catastrophic. The reality is that many of our medications do not offer much benefit but do impact significantly on the ability of an individual to think and function. In desperation to maintain their independence, however, patients are often put on opiate therapy which then causes further problems in the form of constipation, addiction, dependence and withdrawal, together with the suppression of the immune system and cognitive decline.

*

We walk a difficult line in anaesthetics and in the practice of critical care medicine. Ours is not to judge whether prolonging life versus a natural death should be the preferred choice. I once asked a surgeon who operates on people who have cancer of the food pipe what he would do if he was diagnosed with the condition. His response was, 'I would have a stent [a metal tube] placed into my food pipe to keep it open and I would go back home and drink myself to death.' His response is an acknowledgement of the suffering that patients sometimes undergo when having major surgery for cancer of the oesophagus.

In the Western world we work at the very edges of medicine, operating on individuals where the margins between quality of life and incurring suffering are blurred. I have found that in the UK, as opposed to South Africa where I was born and worked for a little while, the attitude is very different in terms of medical intervention. In South Africa if somebody had an illness that you didn't have the ability to manage without heroic efforts then you could say to the family that they should take the relative home to care for them whilst they are dying. This was met with acceptance. In the UK there is often the expectation that people will have every available therapy before shuffling off this mortal coil. It is difficult to know why levels of acceptance surrounding healthcare differ so much between places and cultures. It may reflect the differing availability of resources between countries. It may be cultural; that a belief in an afterlife or ancestors facilitates greater acceptance of death. It may even be due to differing approaches to family structures; I have sometimes found that the relatives who push most for continued treatment appear to not have the best relationship with the patient. Perhaps they yearn for more time to make amends.

Sometimes I wonder how my last days will be, and as I watch some of my patients gradually fade away I wonder about the ethics of prolonging life at the expense of suffering. Pain management in older adults is complex and these ethical conundrums cannot be avoided – although in the West we have a tendency to avoid confronting them. As our medical abilities and technologies continue to develop we are increasingly going to be faced with this dilemma, and it is crucial that we approach it from a well thought out and moral standpoint. I anaesthetized a patient just yesterday with inoperable large bowel cancer and who was having his stoma (the opening in his abdomen through which he now defecated) refashioned. When I asked him if he was okay when he woke up from the anaesthetic his response was, 'No – why did you not just let me go...'

Show me the money – private pain practice

'We are such stuff as dreams are made on, and our little
life is rounded with a sleep.'

The Tempest, Act 4, Scene 1, William Shakespeare

I visit Cape Town on a regular basis to see my parents
and siblings – my brother is a GP and has a little boy
who associates my visits with Lego and my sister is an
academic clinical psychologist. Over the last twenty years
I have watched Cape Town change, becoming an international city where you can have anything your heart desires.
It has become a playground for the rich and famous, with
the advantages and disadvantages that accompany this.
The city centre and surrounding area from the slopes of
Table Mountain to the Atlantic Boardwalk has been rede-
veloped and transformed into a bohemian, hipster and
coffee-lover's paradise. Areas that have been settled for
centuries have now become gentrified and those without
money have slowly been squeezed away from neighbour-
hoods like the Cape Malay area on the slopes of Signal Hill,

moving further and further away from the playgrounds in the city.

There is a bakery where I like to have breakfast which has a seating area where you can simultaneously have a view of Lion's Head and the city framed by the edge of Table Mountain. A short distance from this coffee shop is a very subdued and elegant building. I usually see a couple of Porsches and a Maserati parked outside and if you look at the building's signage it lists as some of its occupants a cosmetic dentist, the rooms of several plastic surgeons, skin-care rejuvenation specialists and dietitians. The building also contains a specialized gym. The men and women who wander into these buildings are already quite beautiful. What I find very interesting about buildings like this (and I have seen them in many parts of the world) is that they very seldom contain the rooms of a group of clinical psychologists.

We live in a world of hashtags and Instagram streaks (apparently the length of successive posts which you are awarded 'likes' for, as I was informed by one of my colleagues who has teenagers) and we have developed technologies to lift, puff, tuck and freeze various parts of our anatomy. On any given news feed the lives of people whose sole occupation seems to be their appearance occupy the same amount of space as stories about corruption, food shortage and war.

We aggressively pursue technological solutions to our inevitable decline and place a premium on external experience that supersedes reason, combined with an impatience that makes us unwilling to embrace the appropriate amount of sleep, correct diet, mindfulness as a virtue and consistency of behaviour to ensure well-being even though we have centuries of spiritual and philosophical guidance that indicate this is the most effective way to lead a long and contented life.

The documentaries that are made about centenarians from the island of Okinawa and in parts of Europe as well as in the US (often Mormons) all indicate that moderation, social cohesion, physical activity and a sense of community are what facilitate longevity. Perhaps, though, we, much like James Dean, would rather crash and burn than fade away – we tend, however, to not have good-looking corpses. The pursuit of perceived perfection and well-being makes us very vulnerable to promises of instantaneous fixes but also at risk of a new type of pain. The experience of pain is an ancient biological alarm system that warns us of real or perceived danger, telling us that we are about to be injured or that we have been injured, and is hardwired into the most primitive parts of our brain. But ultimately the perception of what is harmful is a matter of our own psychological disposition towards the threat or stimulus (having your bottom pinched by your husband or wife is different from that inflicted by a random stranger – same stimulus, different threat interpretation) and therefore exists on a continuum for people. I imagine that the everyday feedback from the body of a professional rugby player, battered by their daily exercise regime and high-intensity games, is not something that the rest of us would put up with, because there would be no context for it. Not having a six-pack when we look down at our stomachs does not leave most of us distressed, but for a cover-page model the experience would be truly frightening. This discomfort from our perception of what is and is not appropriate in terms of how our bodies feel or look leads us to seek help. The manner and method by which we seek help are dictated and modified by the culture we come from and by the explanations and expectations that we have of illness.

We have, in the twenty-first century, beautiful hospitals resplendent with technological marvels including imaging devices that can delineate with stunning clarity the inner architecture of your body. We have sharp needles and processes to obtain blood from patients which are tested in laboratories using spectrophotometers. We have doctors and nurses and occupational therapists and physiotherapists – a veritable armada of people to manage healthcare. Hospitals have managers and accountants and marketing departments; they are now like multifaceted temples or shopping malls for various conditions, and in these vast complexes lies the vested interest of a host of people to maintain the idea that we, the healthcare professionals, are omniscient and omnipotent in terms of helping you live well and live longer.

The often undisclosed reality, however, is that once a society has moved beyond violence in the streets in the form of shooting and stabbings, once people have ceased clubbing each other over the head, and if you live in a home that has a flushing toilet and have access to soap and water on a regular basis as well as appropriate nutrition, then you have probably already saved yourself from around 90 per cent of the maladies that could affect you and for which you would need a hospital. If your car has airbags, you drive slowly and you monitor the age of the car, if everybody follows the rules of the road and observes their stopping distance, then you have probably already accounted for most of that trauma which is not related to interpersonal violence. If you do not drink alcohol (*The Lancet* has now published the evidence that there is no safe limit on alcohol) and therefore avoid subsequently falling down and fracturing your ribs, which accounts for a significant number of hospital admissions in our Trust, and you avoid sugar, which is the new fat, and exercise on a regular basis, then it is likely you need never darken the door of a hospital or your GP. If you love and live mindfully in the moment rather than living in the future where you will become anxious or in the past which will make you depressed, and you maintain your interpersonal relationships and have a clear idea of how you want to live your life, whether that be in service to others or a spiritual belief that you are here to earn an afterlife, then it is likely that you will not trouble our psychologists. The only role left for healthcare then is genetic conditions over which you have no control, or cancers that are manifest as a result of your abnormal genes.

The best thing you can do to not end up in either an overloaded public medical institution, or in a privately paying institution, is to preserve your psychological and musculoskeletal health. This is more easily said than done because we live in a hypocritical world where we tell people to eat less fat and sugar but then supermarkets have aisles and aisles dedicated to crisps and chocolate. We make fruit and vegetables horrendously expensive and we sell cheap, energy-rich but nutritionally poor products such as refined bread and pasta which those on lower incomes have to rely on in place of fresh fruit and vegetables to bulk out their diets. We promote and denigrate in equal measure the meat industry and the dairy industry. We confuse everyone with regards to whether you should or should not drink milk; is dairy good for you or is dairy bad for you? Should you embrace veganism, or will this diet cause a vitamin B12 deficiency? Should you eat more plants? How much protein do you need? We do not make it easy for people to answer these questions. And of course, ultimately there is no diet that guarantees immortality. Even as we become increasingly obsessed with well-being there is a rise in people suffering from disabling chronic pain.

As a society we are seeing a growth in chronic pain, aided and abetted by sugary inactivity and nihilism. There is seldom talk of chronic pain as an epidemic, but that is what we are facing. There is little made of the role that a biopsychosocial approach to the management of chronic pain could play in our society, and no recognition for the work that should be done by healthcare providers in improving the overall health of the population, for example by reducing the consumption of sugar and encouraging more of a focus on exercise and mental well-being. I often reflect on the paradox of our existence – as a society we have the science to support the huge benefits of not eating refined sugar but continue to sell it. We know we should exercise more and be active and yet have invented binge-watching box sets as a sport. What underlies these contradictions? Perhaps we don't consider ourselves worthy of saving, leading to this apathy towards our own decline? Or perhaps it is more existential: because we have the ability to contemplate our mortality we adopt the YOLO (You Only Live Once) approach, wanting the easy things in life and disregarding anything that requires more effort or a longer-term investment. When we then inevitably break, we are not willing to take responsibility ourselves and instead adopt the 'fix me, Doctor' approach. In turn, the doctor who earns his living by fixing you is not incentivized to help you change your lifestyle, which would cut off a source of his income.

The pursuit of well-being is sought through medical intervention, rather than by a shift, both societal and individual, in behaviour and lifestyle. This has inevitably led to an increase in private medical practice. I work in a public sector organization which is funded by the taxpayer. I have therefore been trained at the expense of the taxpayer to offer to those who need them therapies that are grounded in safety, appropriateness, fiscal neutrality and efficacy, and these therapies are free at the point of contact. I am, however, moderated and managed in terms of what I can offer the taxpayer through the assessment, by organizations such as NICE or Clinical Commissioning Groups made up of local GPs, of which therapies are useful and demonstrate benefit based on the available scientific evidence. This was not always the situation and just forty years ago doctors were able to offer therapies which 'in their hands' were considered successful.

Archie Cochrane was a Scottish doctor and is considered the father of clinical epidemiology and evidence-based medicine; in 1979 he wrote, 'It is surely a great criticism of our profession that we have not organized a critical summary, by speciality and subspecialty, adapted periodically, of all randomized controlled trials.' Since then, the autonomy of doctors to make it up as they go along has been gradually curtailed through the implementation of evidence-based practice, which is also sometimes used to restrict therapies as populations explode and governments become poorer. I have just received an email which says that the local commissioning group is stopping the provision of facet joint injections for patients; overnight it has been decreed that we can no longer provide a therapy that we have been offering for thirty years. There are cohorts of patients who will now have to learn to adjust to a new reality where they have no access to this therapy.

Not so if you have access to private healthcare.

If you are willing to pay you will find a doctor who will be able to offer you the procedure you are seeking. But this system is not without its flaws. I heard an orthopaedic surgeon state during a lecture he was delivering to trainee orthopaedic surgeons that the threshold for offering a patient a view of the inside of their knee (an arthroscopy) is based on the same symptoms but varies to a huge degree depending on whether they are an NHS or private patient. The impatience of the privately insured to get better rapidly, combined with the fee earned by the surgeon, reduces the threshold at which intervention is offered. Insurers that offer private healthcare are becoming more savvy to the discrepancies between public and private healthcare, ensuring that they are aware of what is available through the NHS and consequently restricting the services that they are willing to pay for, limiting them to something closer to what is provided to the general public. This is ostensibly in line with the evidence that dictates what services are available on the NHS, but it is also an excellent way of reducing what the patient is offered. I know of a pain medicine consultant who used to inject the patient's lumbar facet joints on their private insurance three times (which was the maximum allowed by the insurance company) before referring the patient to himself to continue the therapy within the NHS.

There is a prevalence in pain medicine these days of pain physicians who are no longer funded to perform procedures in their own country promoting these procedures abroad in places with less regulation. I often see on social media sites that doctors from the UK are going abroad to Dubai and to India, offering courses on X-ray- and ultrasound-guided injections, which are not funded by the NHS for chronic pain. These social media posts are usually accompanied by a photo of a group of smiling individuals gathered around in a lab having learnt a cadaveric approach to an interventional pain procedure, and talk about international collaboration in these countries to promote injection therapies for chronic pain. It is almost as if a scorched Earth policy is being adopted where the fact that these interventions are no longer being offered in the home country has caused a shift to greener pastures, in this case to countries that are somewhat behind in terms of their musculoskeletal epidemics, to offer them the therapies that we now no longer perform because we have realized that they do not serve any purpose in improving function, pain or reducing disability. We are therefore exporting our technical expertise but not our clinical experience or public health destination. These unproven, or even disproven, therapies are simply shifted to countries that have now started to experience their own epidemics of musculoskeletal problems related to living a first-world lifestyle – for a price.

*

Private practice requires individuals to buy private health insurance, which is in itself expensive. This has led to a divide between London and the rest of the UK, following the economic divide, with private practice far less prevalent outside of the capital. Consequently, private hospitals have not developed to the same degree, particularly outside London, and broadly speaking private medicine is not usually as well set up as NHS hospitals for major surgery. In the NHS you will be allocated to a hospital specializing in your surgery, where you will have a tier of on-call health professionals consisting of trainees and, these days, often a consultant. We run a service at our hospital where there is a consultant anaesthesiologist available 24/7 to provide consultant delivered care to the sickest patients. We have fully staffed critical-care units and the laboratory facilities to manage these challenging cases. This is not usually the case in private hospitals in the UK. In South Africa the situation is very different, and the private sector is probably better developed than its public sector counterparts. Money talks, and it speaks very loudly.

A friend of mine told me that their mother had been referred to a rheumatologist in the private sector in South Africa with back pain the other day and on the next day received lumbar facet joint injections. Not only was the injection not logical or supported by the scientific evidence and a thorough assessment of the patient's problem was not made, but the intervention was performed using a CT scanner. This is a completely unnecessary and over-the-top intervention using an imaging technique that we would not use on a routine basis in the UK. But if you do perform the procedure in this way then you can charge for the radiologist's time and thus help fund the purchase of that CT scanner by the hospital. The aim of private hospitals and private medicine is to generate an income for the doctor and for the hospital providing the facility. Unfortunately, patients often approach private hospitals as if they were churches where the benefit to the patient was assured and where the belief is that the people working there are motivated purely by a desire to be of service. I am sure these hospitals and doctors aim to provide excellent healthcare, but ultimately there is a conflict of interest when an institution is being paid for every procedure, plaster and needle used.

The medical records of patients whom I review in the context of a medicolegal claim often reflect on their interaction with pain medicine consultants who they have seen on a private basis. It becomes patently clear that the only way you make any money in private medicine is if you offer patients a procedure. A conversation about chronic pain, an explanation that the pain is due to altered nerve function, and that the aim of pain management is to help the patient start moving more despite continued pain, is not going to get you paid. What gets you paid is offering the patient an injection of local anaesthetic and steroid (every three months) or offering to burn their nerves for a small fee.

I have on many occasions considered taking on a private practice in pain medicine. We have surgeons at our hospital who offer private operations and who sometimes require a pain physician to manage those patients who go on to develop persistent pain. I have visited several of these hospitals, but I have never been able to see a way of replicating what I can offer through the NHS. From a financial point of view, it makes little sense in a private hospital to run a clinic where all you are doing is giving advice, given that the income generator is the delivery of a procedure. The remuneration from a clinic appointment does not cover the extra indemnity that one has to pay to your medical insurer. There is always the fear that in order to cover costs your clinical practice in the private sector will change ever so slightly compared to your NHS practice, becoming more invasive than you would normally be within the NHS. I don't believe that I am an angel, immune to the lure of private practice with its social media marketing and bevy of adoring, grateful and passive middle-class patients, and I might potentially be tempted, albeit subconsciously, to be swayed in this way. And so I have always vacillated when it comes to private practice.

I have tried to start a private practice within the setting of my hospital, but this has not been supported by the hospital management. This reflects one of the great difficulties of working in the NHS. Public sector organizations are not designed to aggressively increase revenue, unlike private hospitals. Hospital management does not therefore have the same approach to increasing and expanding services that a private sector establishment is geared towards. I am often frustrated when trying to implement anything new within the NHS. The first response is always: we have never done that; this is not how we do things. A private practice delivered alongside my NHS work would represent the best of both worlds in the sense that I would be able to give private patients more rapid access to NHS therapies that are not currently offered in private practice, such as neuromodulation and pain management programmes, within the context of the usual safe and clean environment where I work. This would not disadvantage NHS patients, who would still receive these therapies after the usual wait, but would increase the utilization of the theatre and clinic space out of hours, thereby increasing government revenue.

It could be argued that in the provision of healthcare everybody should have access to the same kinds of help based on need and in terms of how adversely they are being affected by a condition rather than because they can pay. One of the aspects of private pain medicine that has always distressed me is that those patients who are willing to pay for a consultation with a pain physician are often the most desperate. They are usually the most psychologically distressed, anxious and depressed patients who catastrophize to a high degree about their pain. They are willing to pay to jump the queue in order to receive a magical cure for their persistent pain and will throw money at the problem in order to resolve their predicament. These patients usually benefit the least from interventional techniques but are the most likely to agitate for them. They are fish in a barrel when it comes to private practice. Unfortunately, when you explain to these patients that there is no cure for their symptoms, they are the most likely to become angry, not just because of their condition but because of the money that they have spent. The temptation in that situation is to offer them an injection therapy in order to quell their rising anger and your resulting distress.

To me, private pain practice represents yet another one of these industries where people with too much money or sometimes too much desperation are willing to go. The doctor has a societal position that enables them to offer a therapy, but they can walk away from it when the treatment doesn't work. I know somebody who has had bilateral knee replacements but continues to be disabled because they have not lost any weight; they have no improvement in function because their underlying behaviour has not changed. The person who has performed the surgery and the person who anaesthetized the patient, however, have benefitted from offering this procedure, as the patient was in a position to pay for it to be done privately. I wonder sometimes about the ethics of saying to somebody, 'I can offer you this procedure but there is no guarantee that it will help you – but if you want it then let's go ahead.' At what point does our responsibility begin and end with regards to performing unnecessary surgery on people? Or is it the case that in a liberal society people can have whatever they ask for if they are willing to accept the risks? I suppose it speaks to a deeper question of whether we operate as individuals or as a global society. It strikes me sometimes that we are racing into oblivion as a species by not taking individual responsibility for our acts.

I have already alluded to my belief that pain medicine is an endangered specialty in the UK, and that its practitioners are increasingly finding that the medical services they provide are being stripped away. Eventually, if you no longer have anything to offer a hospital in terms of generating revenue, then the hospital will tell you to either go away or do something that it does need you for. This is the reality of medical practice – perhaps more obviously in private practice but also underlying in publicly provided services – that it is a business, with financial interests, and the patient is the product.

The beginning of the end

'Now this is not the end. It is not even the beginning of
the end. But it is, perhaps, the end of the beginning.'

Winston Churchill

This final chapter finds me on the Atlantic seaboard
in Cape Town on a Sunday morning sitting directly
across from Robben Island, once a prison, now a
tourist attraction and a stark reminder of the inhumanity
that we can display towards one another, entrenched in law
and justified by the selective interpretation of a religious
text. It is a grey morning in Cape Town – Signal Hill and
Table Mountain are still covered with stubborn clouds and
are not yet visible, and the sea is more suited to being pho-
tographed in noir than technicolour.

The boardwalk which snakes from the Waterfront is a
hive of physical and meditative activity. Some early risers
stare out to sea, lost in thought, whilst others pound the
pavement in colourful Lycra sometimes stretched beyond
breaking point and sometimes embracing the athletic
forms that it was designed to serve. Some runners move

lithely, in perfect rhythm with bodies that display efficient power-to-weight ratios and the flexibility needed to chase their food – as if they were designed to run; others trundle along with minimal hip movement, knees groaning, and all I can think about is the blank cheques that are being written to hospitals and the future expansion of the bank balances of orthopaedic surgeons, as these runners slowly and, it appears, painfully grind away at the front part of their knees. Their dogs run around them, occasionally interested in their owner's progress and now and then staring up at them wondering what the purpose of the run is because it clearly is not in pursuit of breakfast. Other Capetonians have decided that two wheels represent far better exercise and speed by in a blur of carbon fibre. The common thread is a pursuit of health and well-being; the form this takes is based on each individual's selective exposure to and inter-pretation of the information bombarding them.

If you have reached this point in the book, then you have seen through my eyes – sometimes clear and sometimes jaundiced but always, I hope, open and curious. This book about pain reflects the last twenty-two years of my journey and career which started on the slopes of Devil's Peak at the University of Cape Town, moved to the far north of South Africa before a series of placements in the UK, in Plymouth, Warwick, Swindon, Bath and finally ending up in Manchester and Salford. It is my journey of working in places ranging from those where human life means little and interpersonal violence is rife, to places where extending life is of supreme importance – sometimes beyond what is reasonable, achievable or kind. From hospitals where we barely had enough equipment to hospitals where over-investigation is the order of the day. This book reflects my personal journey, from not wanting to engage with people and preferring them to be anaesthetized when I work with them, to a place where the greatest joy and satisfaction has been derived from long-term relationships with patients and their families.

Alongside my own story, I have tried to provide an overview of the history of pain and our understanding of this phenomenon over time. What has become clear to me as I have written this book is that human beings have always been afflicted with pain – that we are creatures that are intimate with suffering and mindful of our decline and eventual end. We live such short lives and cower in the face of eternity, desperately engaged in immortality projects – children, money, fame and the accumulation of stuff. In my view this short lifespan gives us a unique but quite distorted perspective of ourselves and where we fit in to the span of human history; we rarely have the opportunity to witness change over even a hundred years. Perhaps that's why we repeat the same mistakes again and again – or perhaps it is because we cling to hope, left in Pandora's infamous box not as a boon but as a curse for humanity.

In a week's time it will have been twenty years since I graduated from medical school, and whilst I can remember elements of the last twenty years, and if you asked me to recall specific events I can, much of the detail is lost to me.

The moments that are most memorable are those associated with the greatest pain, and not in a purely negative way – the greatest discomfort and times of discord have also been the greatest moments of learning and progress. We like to think that our choices are made in the fullness of joy and in moments of quiet reflection brought on by contentment, but the truth is that as a species we often make dramatic steps forward when we are most uncomfortable. We therefore have a relationship with pain and suffering which is characterized not just by negativity but also by complexity and growth.

Pain has always been in the background, and sometimes in the foreground, of our evolution as a species. When we were single-cell organisms our only responses were those towards growth or away from pain. Even in our highly evolved state today, pain is still a teacher – the discomfort of emotional and physical adversity and injury prompts learning: don't touch that, don't go there, wear sunblock, don't date narcissists. We have fast pain fibres that get us out of trouble and slow pain fibres that result in any persistent unpleasantness laying down a memory of the event and teaching us to avoid that which caused us harm. Sometimes we accept discomfort and pain, viewing it as an experience that we need to endure in order to grow – pain following a gym session is accepted based on the belief that muscles will improve as a result. The report of pain always has context – in some situations inflicting harm is experienced as fifty shades of pleasure.

Perhaps our narrative with regards to the experience of pain is also shaped by our ability from a technological point of view to influence the experience. When there was nothing that we could do to alleviate pain, our way of assuaging the experience was to believe that it was necessary. When treating pain became something that we actively and passionately sought to do, because we now understand the disease and know of a treatment, then our enthusiasm has known no bounds and our philosophy has become that it is inhumane not to manage pain. I wonder if this has less to do with pain and more to do with the structure and nature of our societies; our modern society values the individual and treating the pain of the individual has therefore become an essential part of the human narrative.

Our technology continues to evolve, and our understanding of the neurobiology of pain evolves alongside the scientific tools increasingly available to study it. But in my view, we are still very much looking from the outside in, desperately feeling around to try to understand what this phenomenon is. I think what separates pain from many other symptoms is that it is so intimately tied into how we interpret the world. Diarrhoea is pretty much diarrhoea. It has a beginning and an end and if we can find a cause then hopefully we can return our bowel function to normal. The nature of pain, however, is that it completely commands our attention – it is 'aversive at threshold', to return to our opening definition. Pain activates brain areas that are primitive and archaic, present from when we were unicellular organisms; it sits alongside the need for food, the compulsion to procreate and the irresistible pull of sleep, in this ancient brain. Pain is a constant life companion, present not just physically but also psychologically and emotionally. I believe that trying to understand and treat an experience like pain cannot be separated from trying to understand and manage people.

Having said this, ultimately understanding pain as a disease and then being able to target the molecular basis of pain is probably a better way forward than trying to ignore pain, distract yourself from it and therefore live well despite persistent pain. Pain is, after all, a primitive and hardwired alarm whose purpose is to warn that all is not well, and eventually we hope to be able to switch the alarm system off in the same way we hope to *cure* diabetes with stem cells rather than *managing* it by giving insulin. However, we do not currently have the understanding or capabilities to tackle pain in this way, and trying to treat the experience of pain is what we are left with due to our limited understanding of pain and our suboptimal therapies.

Our medical understanding is constantly progressing; today, for example, in many respects we understand cancers that once mystified us. Pain is sometimes a manifestation of a cancerous condition (although not always) and in such cases we treat the underlying cancer in order to prolong life, arresting those cells which have gone rogue as best we can with instruments which in a hundred years will probably seem quite primitive. In doing so, we poison the abnormal cell, but we also taint the healthy cell alongside it. We irradiate both healthy and unhealthy cells and we cut out and brutally destroy the malfunctioning cancerous mass whilst trying to preserve the normal tissue. We understand the pain which accompanies cancer. We understand it because we believe it to be due to a disease that we comprehend. And yet, patients with identical tumours can experience vastly different levels of pain, and we must therefore accept that even this apparently understood process is interpreted through an individual's unique cognitive, behavioural and emotional framework.

We understand the immediate pain associated with damaged tissues. That is to say, we at least understand the source, but we do not always appreciate the variability. Understanding *why* somebody has pain is much easier than trying to understand how they feel and how they suffer. In seeking to provide medical treatment, as doctors we inflict pain daily – we damage tissues and then try to repair, reconstruct and reformulate. We hope that in our destruction we achieve a measure of improvement – in function or in longevity – but pain is sometimes the inevitable consequence of that endeavour. We try to dampen it down for as long as is needed for tissues to heal and stop crying out against the insult that they have endured. Whilst doing this we try not to poison the patient with medications that may cause addiction and worsen their outcome or cause bleeding from their stomachs or damage their nerves with needles that we place in order to deposit local anaesthetic.

Where we struggle most is when our current technology is unable to identify the source of pain. People who present with pain in a part of their bodies where modern technology is unable to identify anything that is broken or cancerous are viewed with suspicion. In the past we have consigned patients like this to asylums. Patients who were sent to asylums with seizure activity in the nineteenth century were found later to have brain tumours in about 60 per cent of cases. More recently, we have tried to manage the patient's behaviour by sedating them with opioids or damaging normal parts of their nervous system in order to quieten down the alarm that has been blaring. We have injected, electrocuted, tranquilized and psychologized this group of patients because our technology is unable to diagnose the dysfunction which is causing them to cry out in pain. These patients are generally referred to by doctors as heart-sink patients. They are caught in a vortex of misunderstanding and are not helped by a system that is designed to support the management of specific, identifiable conditions. We find it hard to accept that there are patients where we have to say to them, 'I have done all the tests that we currently have at our disposal. These tests have not shown me anything in your organs that I can cure. We do not yet understand why some people develop conditions like yours. There are treatments, but they are designed to be empiric and there is no evidence that they will improve your function or reduce your pain but there is a high probability that they will turn you into an addict or that they will damage parts of your body that are functioning normally. You are not mad, and you are not imagining the symptoms – it is just that we do not yet have the ability to diagnose your condition with a scan or a blood test.'

One of the most difficult emotional situations that doctors find themselves in is when they have to communicate the explanation above. When you talk about a pain which science cannot measure, most patients end up believing that you are telling them that the problem is all in their heads – the question 'Why is it that we can put a man on the moon but we cannot cure my pain?' has been uttered in clinic more than once in my career. Unfortunately, the fact is that we do not have the ability to analyse nervous system function at any more than an electrophysiological level, which measures gross conduction of electrical activity in nerves. Our ability to image the nervous system is confined to that of an MRI scan, and whilst we do have some tests that can measure blood flow in the brain in response to different stimuli, these tests are not yet specific enough to accurately diagnose a 'cause' for many pain conditions.

*

I used to think very narrowly about pain, viewing it through the lens of a subspecialist in terms of just managing the person's pain. I realize now that people exist in a context. Patients do not come to the pain clinic with just their pain. They may talk about only their pain, but they come with many psychological difficulties related to other life events and sometimes horrific social circumstances that you are completely unaware of until you read the letter generated by the psychologist. Patients are usually but not always overweight due to a poor diet; sometimes this is because of a lack of education, or they may eat to comfort themselves and eating becomes a way of coping. Patients may overuse alcohol as a means of coping, and may then use prescription opiates in a similar manner; opiates become their new vodka. The aim with these patients is not so much to treat the pain but to treat the associated distress and despair, which in some way ameliorates the pain.

When I talk to patients now in clinic I am much more aware of their hidden context and shadow selves. I explain pain to them as best I can, and try to encourage an understanding of chronic pain. I don't want people to leave my clinic thinking that the pain is all in their head but I do want them to understand that they have the ability to influence the abnormal sensations they are experiencing. I try to help them understand that every aspect of their lives influences their pain, and that is what we need to tackle. Their diets, for instance, are a manifestation of their distress but also contribute to perpetuating the condition. We often focus on the external manifestation of a behavioural problem or a maladaptive thought pattern more than we do on the actual thought or behaviour, but both need addressing simultaneously. As I commented in the previous chapter, there were no psychologists in the beautiful grey building under the mountain. If there was a psychologist on the first floor, whom you had to see first, then it is likely you would only progress to the levels above if there was an identifiable physiological problem; you would only see the dentist if your teeth required treating and you would only see the skincare specialist if you actually had a dermatological condition. It is unlikely that you would ever make it to the floor occupied by the cosmetic surgeons.

As part of my clinic I explain the current dietary recommendations that should be followed, as well as discussing how psychological wellness is predicated around a clear understanding of thoughts and feelings and that people need to find a reason for living and a meaning to their existence. It might be argued that I am exceeding my scope of practice as a pain clinician, but my view is that we shouldn't really be called a pain clinic, we should be called a wellbeing clinic. It strikes me that any doctor that you visit should have this approach to a patient's wellness. Rather than focusing on inserting another stent into their coronary arteries they should reflect on why, in the three years since they put the last stent in, the patient has not made any changes to modify their risk factors. By not being this sort of doctor, are we not culpable of continuing our own middle-class pursuit of healthcare?

I have not even mentioned smoking or recreational drug taking because to me these pursuits seem so obviously harmful, but the very fact that these substances still exist and are readily available speaks volumes about our paradoxical attitudes to our own health. We continue to promote cigarettes even though we say that smoking kills on the packaging. We bemoan the impact of soft drinks on the health of the population, particularly those on lower incomes, but then we continue to manufacture these substances. We of course also eschew and decry wars all over the world but then continue to produce armaments. I often reflect quite sadly that in many areas of the world where there is conflict, those areas do not actually have factories producing the weapons themselves; I then wonder whether if the countries manufacturing them stopped providing guns, eventually they would get tired of fighting with sticks and stones. Perhaps because we are the only species that is able to understand that we will die, we sometimes in our despair rush towards self-destruction.

*

Pain medicine is not a pursuit that I would necessarily choose to return to in another life. I think that modern medicine is pretty good at treating injuries. I often fantasize that if I were to come back as a healthcare professional in the next life I would be an orthopaedic surgeon treating trauma victims. The bone is broken, and I can fix it – this is a simple interaction with the patient from an architectural point of view. Disruption or discontinuity to the normal anatomical structures because they are physically traumatized is something that one can easily repair, theoretically.

Pain on the other hand is a complex experience and it is not one over which we have mastery, either where it has been triggered due to injury or where it has become persistent in the case of chronic pain. In the acute setting we can manage the underlying or precipitating condition. We can remove the drawing pin from your foot and clean the wound and apply a plaster. We can put plates and screws on your broken bone and make sure the tissues do not become infected. We can treat your burns to a certain extent by putting dressings on them or taking away the dead tissue. We can treat your chemical injury appropriately. We can give you medications in the form of anti-inflammatories or local anaesthetics or morphine until the nervous system's alarm settles down.

Where you have persistent pain all over your body because of an accumulated lifetime of psychological and immunological injury caused by adopting a reckless lifestyle or a psychosocially poor environment, we do not have a medical cure for this pain. Where you have developed persistent pain because you are too heavy for your knees – this is where we struggle. If you have damaged a nerve in your body through injury and whilst the nerves have healed the pain has not resolved, we are less adept at managing your pain. Even therapies such as spinal cord stimulation which appear to be quite sophisticated to us today, may be considered barbaric a hundred years from now.

I have become increasingly despondent over the last few years about my role as a healthcare professional. I sometimes feel that I am colluding with my colleagues, caught in a system that operates on the margins, with an understanding of pain that is no better than we had a hundred years ago. Pain medicine is one of the specialties where we have created an entire industry based on the most inexcusably weak base of evidence. We are now being found out and government bodies responsible for allocating healthcare resources are uncovering the waste of resources that have been ploughed into injection therapies that have not been appropriately studied.

The most powerful and therapeutic part of my role as a healthcare professional is to explain pain. It is the only tool at my disposal which, in my experience, makes a difference to patients. Even when patients are angry and disappointed when informed that their condition is permanent and that the alarm system will never return to normal, the mere introduction to an approach acknowledging that there is no cure is in itself the start of a healing process. Most patients will continue on the roundabout of medical investigations and treatment but at least at some point somebody has said to them 'this is a permanent condition and we do not yet have the answer'. Unfortunately, as an industry, healthcare can take a glib view of pain, and most people are never exposed to an understanding from a healthcare physician about the complexity of pain. In most medical schools pain is given mere lip service as an experience. It is simply the introduction to the more interesting diagnosis using our latest technology and a very short period of foreplay before the main event of treatment.

Healthcare and medicine require, in my opinion, a fundamental rethink in terms of where we are heading. Archie Cochrane asked us to collect and systematize the evidence base for what we do; this has been done in many specialties, but there is still a deep need to then implement, study and improve on these therapies. Independent bodies are needed to look at where we are currently in terms of treatment and to design rational therapies without collusion with industry (my dream is to trial a spinal cord stimulator system manufactured without a brand name, one which is able to offer all stimulation parameters within a single system). We need to accept that many of the aspects of modern life are damaging to people, and that merely providing passive solutions from a healthcare point of view is at best futile and at worst unethical. We understand how to prevent a huge number of diseases but invest very little in actually doing so because, ultimately, we profit from the managing of conditions which people inflict upon themselves, aided and abetted by society's marketing of the modern lifestyle.

Being a doctor today is complex and I often feel inadequate in my role, with the pills and potions at my disposal often hailing from ancient times and simply repackaged for the twenty-first century. I feel that we have lost our way in medicine and are desperately searching for a way back in order to justify our worth. In the UK we have few infectious diseases, cars travel relatively slowly, and gun ownership is almost non-existent; I treat diseases of lifestyle and the ravages of time. Why are we not more involved in the primary prevention of disease?

Medicine continues to be a middle-class pursuit and there are significant issues with where we draw medical students from in terms of reflecting the wider society. There is also the concern that, over time, those who enter medicine become more interested in maintaining their role than in changing society. Whilst it is not always the case, I think that holding on to a perceived degree of wealth and position in society is what motivates some doctors in terms of the way that they practise medicine. When you combine this with the potential rewards available in private practice then in certain healthcare systems around the world you end up with a situation where people are exploited and are subjected to unnecessary investigations, tests and procedures. Patients sometimes actively collude with doctors in that there can be a significant psychological pay-off for them in terms of adopting the sick role, again facilitated by our modern society.

Who becomes the arbiter of whether somebody should have a procedure depends on the country where you find yourself. Ideally it should be independent institutions – without affiliations to pharmaceutical and technology companies or anything that might lead to their own enrichment – that should decide what is offered and, more importantly, what requires further study, based on the available evidence. Even in a publicly funded system such as the NHS, however, this does not always happen because of lobbying by physicians who are subtly (and not so subtly) sponsored by drug and technology companies and the inherent flaws in many scientific studies.

There also needs to be a shift away from doctors as the primary providers of healthcare and well-being and towards a more global appreciation of the factors that influence health, taking the definition of health put forward by the WHO as a complete state of mental and physical well-being and not merely the absence of disease. The reality is that this requires an abandoning of self-interest on the part of doctors who should first do no harm; those elected to govern should define with evidence the policies that will facilitate well-being and industries should be rewarded for providing therapies that are demonstrated to enhance quality of life. Given the current political climate of the world and the general lack of global cooperation, I am pessimistic about this happening.

One of the great weaknesses in healthcare is that research is difficult to perform and is encumbered by so much administration that most doctors in clinical medicine are put off from participating in it. It is a crime that we are not more actively involved in research as clinicians, but we are so busy offering treatments (which do not always ensure a good outcome) that we are not given the time and space to ask the important questions that need to be asked about the therapies that we offer. Governments are interested in telling patients that they have provided X number of procedures and X number of weeks reduction in waiting times.

What is less sexy is being told that they are investing more in research in order to answer the fundamental questions about what underpins good health. In the UK we can't even organize a meaningful sugar tax and our attempts to reduce alcohol and tobacco consumption are pitiful, even though we know that these recreational activities end up costing society enormous sums – both physically and financially.

For me, continuing to work in a unit that offers pain management physiotherapy and psychology in order to reduce the distress and disability which patients experience due to pain, seems the best and least harmful option for now. Spinal cord stimulation for the management of peripheral neuropathic pain based on strong evidence is a worthy pursuit. Ongoing exploration of the dysfunction that is chronic pain and attempting to design specific therapies to modify this system is a global endeavour. Resisting the empiric use of cannabis oil or cannabis-derived products until clear evidence is established, in the form of randomized controlled trials utilizing these substances in specific pain conditions, is a sure way to prevent this drug from becoming the newest method to medicate despair. Treating existential crises with alcohol, tobacco, cocaine and methamphetamines will clearly not lead to an improved quality of life for the patient. Judicious, kind and measured use of opioids, whilst communicating the risks and benefits of these drugs to the patient, is just. The most important work, however, is to try to explain pain kindly, gently and plainly, based on our current understanding of what pain is and what the limits of treatment are from a medical point of view. Highlighting the aspects of positive living, as found in societies where people live well and for a long time, is essential: whole foods, regular physical activity, living in community with one another and having a shared ideology – finding your *ikigai*, your reason for being.

My hope is that after reading this book you will take responsibility for your health and ask questions of those from whom you seek advice when you are unwell. That when you are in pain you will be able to reflect on the screaming of your primitive brain and understand that the experience of pain is a biological alarm, but your response is a choice. Hopefully you will understand that pain can never be completely extinguished with medicines and can appreciate their potential for harm. Perhaps you will now be able to work with your doctor or nurse when you are in pain. If you have chronic pain, then I hope this book makes you feel acknowledged. If you know someone who suffers with chronic pain, then hopefully you are more informed, which is the soil wherein compassion grows.

In the words of American physician Edward Trudeau, 'Sometimes to cure, often to relieve, always to comfort.'

Acknowledgements

From my patients I have been taught the meaning of Maya Angelou's words: 'I've learned that people will forget what you said, people will forget what you did, but people will never forget how you made them feel.' Thank you for the privilege of being able to serve you.

This book reflects the skill and patience of the people that I work with at the Manchester and Salford Pain Centre who have taught me and whom I continue to learn from.

I would like to thank Dr Tom Mount who put me in touch with Ben Clark from the Soho Agency because he thought I might have something useful to say about pain. Thank you, Ben, for your guidance and encouragement.

Thank you to Katherine Ailes for your thoughtful and kind editing of the manuscript, as well as James Nightingale from Atlantic Books for shaping the finished product.

Index